LITTLE PATIENT BIG DOCTOR

ONE MOTHER'S JOURNEY

HALEH RABIZADEH RESNICK

Copyright © 2010 Haleh Rabizadeh Resnick
All rights reserved.

ISBN: 1452844542
ISBN-13: 9781452844541
Library of Congress Control Number: 2010906336

TABLE OF CONTENTS

ACKNOWLEDGEMENTS ... i

INTRODUCTION ... iii

ETHAN ... 1
- TRADITIONAL MEDICINE: ALLERGISTS AND NUTRITIONISTS ... 29
- PATIENT / DOCTOR COMMUNICATION ... 44
- REIKE ... 46
- MENTAL WELL BEING ... 52
- ONE LAST EFFORT: STEROIDS AND ANTI-BIOTICS ... 61
- DR. DIANNE ... 64
- THE HEALING POTENTIAL ... 69
- ALTERNATIVE DOCTORS ... 70
- NAVIGATING POSSIBILITIES ... 83

ALEX ... 85
- WEEK ONE: WELCOME HOME ... 91
- WEEK TWO: SETTLING IN ... 94
- WEEK THREE: ALADDIN- KIDS CAN'T FLY ... 95
- WEEK FOUR: SUKKOT- LIVE IT UP ... 96

WEEK FIVE: ROCKING THE BOAT … 98

WEEKS SIX – EIGHT: ALL YOU NEED IS YOUR HEALTH … 103

WEEK NINE: NO SLEEP FOR THE WEARY … 104

WEEK TEN: JUST KEEP LIVING … 109

WEEK ELEVEN: DRINKING THE JUICE … 117

THIRD MONTH: CAN YOU HEAR ME? … 120

KEEPING TRACK OF IT ALL … 129

FOURTH MONTH: IT TAKES GUTS … 131

NURTURE YOURSELF: WE NEED EACH OTHER … 144

FIFTH MONTH: THE SECOND OPINION … 146

CONCLUSION … 153

DISCUSSION / READING GROUP QUESTIONS … 155

SOME BOOKS I'VE READ … 157

Acknowledgements

It is my desire that when you finish reading about my journey, you will find the inner strength and courage you need to face any medical issue you or those close to you may have. This book is presented in order to foster a stronger partnership between you and your doctor as you find a way to maximize your healing potential by utilizing both traditional and alternative remedies. Quotations in this book are used stylistically and are not the exact words of speakers.

Helping each other is a team effort. There are many who I would like to thank.

Thank you to my editor, Cindy Silvert, who encouraged me and lent her expertise to this endeavor.

Thank you to Ben Rabizadeh and David Rabizadeh for their internet and marketing assistance. Thank you to my agent Jeff Resnick for helping make this publication possible.

Thank you to my parents for their guidance, friendship, loving support and continual sacrifices. Thank you to my children for their cooperation and for being excited as I wrote this book. Thank you to my husband, my best friend and partner.

Thank you God for surrounding us with wonderful individuals and blessing us with strength and resources to guide us through our challenges.

May you be blessed likewise.

A portion of the proceeds of this book will be given to charity.

Introduction

Dear Doctor,

I want to share with you my experiences with two of my children.

Ethan is a boisterous, upbeat kid with severe allergies. He has allergic reactions to countless foods, some through ingestion, some by contact and some airborne. He also has environmental allergies and has reactions to chemical products with strong odors. When faced with an allergen, his body's response could be as minor as a few random hives on his skin or as intense as an anaphylactic reaction necessitating immediate emergency intervention.

As a newborn, Alex, who is about three years younger than Ethan, was diagnosed with severe hearing loss in both ears. A number of specialists told us that he would have to wear hearing aids by the time he was six months old in order to have the opportunity to develop normal speech.

Both astonished their doctors with unlikely positive outcomes. My experiences with Ethan and Alex taught me that there are many paths that need to be traveled to find good health.

Doctor, my respect for you comes easily. You studied long and hard to acquire your knowledge of medicine. But it has not been easy working with you. There is a communication gap between us. It seems that the more specialized your skill, the less you look at us as a whole. We are left to research and discover whether any other cause outside of your field of knowledge is contributing to our problem. As patients we have to put all the pieces together by ourselves. These days we have access to so many ways of healing other than pure medical relief. We need to work as partners to incorporate traditional and alternative methods of healing.

Navigating health care issues are challenging. We need your help. I would like my story to allow you to view medical care from a patient's perspective, so that we can work together more effectively.

Thanks for all you do,
Haleh

THIS BOOK IS INTENDED ONLY TO ENCOURAGE AN OVERALL APPROACH TO HEALTH. THE INFORMATION IN THIS BOOK IS NOT INTENDED AS MEDICAL ADVICE.

We are a family. We laugh and love and grow with each other. Each person gives a warmth to our family that is unique. Each person is a vital cog. And like all families there are some rough times.

Ethan

> I am with God, God is with me;
> I have the power and strength of God.
> I am with God, God is with me;
> I have the power and strength of God.
> I am with God, God is with me;
> I have the power and strength of God.

I can't believe this is happening. When I went through labor before, it was paaaaainnnful. This time, though, I am okay.

After the birth of my last child, I hadn't been quite well physically. I had stomach and skin problems and various doctors had not been able to help me. Recently, I tried yoga and "mind over body" exercises to help me heal.

I use this same technique, now, during labor. I can't believe that it actually works. Each contraction hits me with a wave of pressure but just as quickly leaves my body. No pain. The nurses and my husband look at me in amazement. The computer monitor shows the coming contraction that should hit my body like a sledgehammer. But I am in peace. The room is silent as I continue my prayer.

> I am with God, God is with me;
> I have the power and strength of God.
> I am with God, God is with me;
> I have the power and strength of God.
> I am with God, God is with me;
> I have the power and strength of God.

And so, Ethan comes into this world. With a headful of blond hair and fair skin, I couldn't believe he was my child. I have that perpetual tanned skin, which turns black in the summer with long, curly, dark brown hair. His dad on the other hand, well. . . he doesn't have much hair now and what he has is starting to gray. He's dignified- those lucky men- but he was blond as a child. None of my other children were blond but that blond gene finally worked its way out. He looks like an angel too - bet you've never heard a mom say that before.

I always wanted a big family. As a child, I remember watching "The Sound of Music" and the "The Brady Bunch" and loving the bustle of a large family. Thankfully, my husband was on the same page.

When we were still in the hospital, Ethan, like most other babies, was a pleasure. For those first two days, when the nurses are around to help and the baby sleeps in the nursery, having a baby seems like a breeze. Then we come home and the storm hits.

Some people are gifted with a baby who sleeps through the night immediately. Who are those people? Are they telling the truth? Anyway. . . Ethan simply stayed awake. He never slept. Our home was filled with so much activity from his older siblings that we first thought Ethan either did not want to sleep (and miss out on the action) or was not able to sleep due to the commotion – day or night. But at some point we realized that the normal hustle and bustle was not the problem. There was something else going on here. He just didn't seem comfortable.

I nursed Ethan and soon noticed that during most feedings he seemed to be scratching at his throat. I didn't think much of this at first. He just seemed to be a very active baby. But I did notice that he didn't have that beautiful baby skin. He was very red and no matter how low I cut his nails, he always had cuts all over his face. Always one to look at the bright side, even to the point of denial, I told myself that he's just a baby with a few extra scratches on his face.

I was in the pediatrician's office a number of times in that first month. I've had my pediatrician for years. He's one of those self-assured types. He's not exceptionally tall but he takes over the little examining room when he walks in. And along with it he has a wry sense of humor, poking fun at situations he's presented with. He's been at this business for so long, I'm sure he's used the jokes before. I like laughter to break the tension.

After a few weeks, the pediatrician diagnosed Ethan's condition as eczema, which is essentially, dry, itchy, irritated skin. The doctor told me, "Lots of babies have it. It's not a big deal. Just put this steroid cream on him and he'll be fine."

Now, unfortunately, eczema was not new to me. As I mentioned, after my previous child was born, I had various physical ailments, part of which included developing severe eczema and hives. I had been to at least a half a dozen different dermatologists in search of a way to eliminate this condition. All of them recommended topical and if necessary oral steroids to manage the eczema and hives. Steroids work wonders to temporarily heal the skin (and this benefit to the body at times outweighs the harm) but do not address the underlying cause of any skin condition. The eczema simply returns when the steroid use is discontinued. Long-term use of oral steroids can wreak havoc on the body and even short-term use can cause a host of temporary problems, such as ulcers, mood changes, constipation and weight gain.

I didn't like the answers I heard, so I kept looking. I wasn't comfortable with repeated steroid use, the standard medical treatment for eczema, even if it was only topical. When I was pregnant with Ethan, my eczema was so severe that I eventually succumbed to taking oral steroids to control the eczema. This was a pretty drastic measure, but I was desperate and my doctors assured me that after the first trimester it would be safe.

When the pediatrician prescribed steroids for Ethan, I protested, "I don't want to put steroids on him. He's just a baby. Isn't there anything else I can do?"

"Not really. This is what works best. If you keep him moisturized after a bath, that will help, but to really keep it under control, you need the steroid."

On my way home, I dutifully picked up the tube of steroid cream. I called my husband and we convinced ourselves that if the doctor says the topical steroid is safe, then it's okay.

I used it twice a day, as prescribed, and it worked its wonders. Ethan's skin was clear. But my mom's conscience was not.

My mom is an "amateur doctor" with her knowledge coming from the "old country" and constant reading. She is always learning something new and passing it along to us. Her understanding is that medicine, though useful, is not the only way to cure an ailment and is usually not even the best way.

So, steroids on Ethan? Well, that was something to stay away from. Not that I disagreed. Despite all the doctor's assurances that topical steroids are not absorbed systemically into the body, I remember quite well that during my pregnancy there were certain topical steroids that no one wanted me to use. If topical steroids are not absorbed into the body, why the concern during pregnancy? And if there is concern during pregnancy, why did that concern not apply to a newborn? It didn't make sense that the topical use of steroids remained just on the skin and any absorption to the body was negligible.

My mom did not feel comfortable with steroid use. I agreed with her and stopped using the steroid on Ethan. Instead, I started to lather my son with

Vaseline. I figured Vaseline can't do too much harm. His skin actually looked a little better with the Vaseline- sticky but soft. Still, Ethan was not fully comfortable.

At the next month's routine visit, the doctor noted Ethan's eczema. His rosy cheeks weren't a sign of a healthy growing baby, as much as my husband and I wanted to see it that way. They were chapped and irritated.

"Are you using the steroid?" asked the doctor.

"No."

I expressed my concern that the steroids would be absorbed into Ethan's system and wouldn't even cure his underlying condition.

He shook his head and explained that Ethan was just uncomfortable and I was needlessly making him suffer. I had to use the steroids. "Don't worry, it's safe," he told me.

When I asked him why I wasn't supposed to use steroids during pregnancy but could put them on Ethan now, my doctor explained with authority and certainty, "In utero, the baby is still developing.

Once born, the baby is developed and steroid use is safe." What if my child is born premature and not fully developed; is steroid use okay then? And isn't the first few years of a child's life one of intense development and growth? How come steroid use is okay in childhood? He could not answer my questions adequately. He shook his head and told me not to worry so much.

But he couldn't reassure me, so, he sent me home with the names of a few over the counter creams known to relieve eczema as well as another steroid prescription for when I would come to my senses.

At home, I started to test the over the counter creams on Ethan. Some worked very well. I also stopped eating and drinking dairy. I have other children who had been allergic to dairy for their first year of life and thought maybe Ethan was allergic also and the allergy was manifesting itself on his skin. As it turned out, cutting out dairy and using the other creams were helpful- to a point. But unfortunately, Ethan's eczema persisted and his face was continually scratched and irritated.

By Ethan's fourth month visit, my doctor had enough with my limited steroid use. I used steroids on Ethan when his skin was very bad but only occasionally and only until his skin cleared. The doctor did not think that was enough. "This poor baby is suffering," he again told me, and "you need to realize the steroid cream is necessary for his comfort."

No mother wants her baby to suffer. But I thought and felt that the steroid would somehow be more harmful to him. If there was any way to naturally treat the dry skin, I wanted to pursue it.

I asked if Ethan could be allergic to anything.

"No. You are nursing. Nursing babies are not allergic. Mother's milk protects them. Just use the cream, he'll be fine."

It was not easy to listen to the doctor berate me, but I listened because he was the expert. Though I continued to ask my questions and had my doubts, I still heard what the doctor had to say.

And, when he was done telling me I wasn't doing the right thing, I thankfully could see in his face that he had an alternative for me. There was a new drug on the market. It suppressed the immune system in a finer way than steroids. Eczema is partly due to over activity of the immune system. This new topical drug calms an overactive system at an early stage and therefore clears the skin. I just had to apply it to irritated areas, which, we agreed, was essentially Ethan's whole body.

I went to the drug store and bought the drug. I can't explain it. Something about this drug did not feel right. It actually pained me to put it on him. It was such a visceral reaction I can only call it instinct. Not surprisingly, my mother didn't like this either.

"Suppress the immune system? That makes no sense. We have to make him stronger not weaker. We can't suppress his natural system. He'll get sick."

"But mom, the doctor says that his system is overactive."

My mom shook her head. This just made no sense to her.

That did it for me. Two moms against one doctor. Mothers know best. I had to continue searching for a better alternative.

Ethan was becoming an active member of our family but he was not comfortable. He could now sit up and interact with the other children. He was engaged and involved. But he did not sleep well and he did not look well. He cried often and was not at peace. One of my children drew a family picture in which everyone was smiling except for a crying Ethan.

A friend of mine suggested that I carry Ethan in a baby snuggler. She said it helped calm her fussy baby. I tried it. I carried Ethan everywhere. Over sweatshirts and business suits, I carried Ethan in a denim-blue snuggler. I was a cross between a hippie and a trendsetter. On some level it worked. It was the only way I could get him to nap during the day. But he still was not truly comfortable. It was clear that his skin was bothering him.

And as his eczema flared, my skin did the same. We suffered with eczema together.

Both my husband and I have relatives in New York or from New York. For any of you familiar with those who come from New York, you've probably heard that New York is the center of the world. Constantly, we were bombarded with advice to go to New York. The best doctors are there- so we are told. I dismissed this notion for a while but I eventually agreed to bring Ethan to a New York doctor.

I finally agreed because suddenly Ethan's eczema became more severe. His skin was red, blotchy and practically oozing. I couldn't even bare to change his diaper. I didn't want to look at his legs; it just reduced me to a puddle of tears. My other children, after trying to calm me, called my mother on the phone and asked her to come over to change Ethan's diaper.

Have you ever tried to get a dermatologist appointment when you really need one? I couldn't find anything sooner than a month away. Then, an aunt from New York gave my mother her dermatologist's number. My mother called and we had an appointment for the next day.

My father-in-law drove Ethan and me to the appointment; he has the map of the entire country in his head. For anyone else a drive out of town is a source of tension. For him, "No problem. I'll take you. I know a shorter route that avoids all the traffic. Just make sure to be ready at seven thirty-five. If it's five minutes later we'll never get there and five minutes earlier, we'll get there too soon."

The drive was easy and we got there with just the right amount of time to sit in the waiting room for the allotted twenty minutes that all doctors seem to require. As I sat in the waiting room, I found myself actually hoping that maybe New York really is the center of the world and that the doctors there could cure Ethan of his horrible eczema. I had been to several dermatologists for myself and had not had much success- but they weren't in New York.

When it was Ethan's turn, I walked into the examination room filled with hope. And when the tall gentleman, with the firm handshake, deep voice and white doctor's jacket arrived, I thought for a moment maybe he knows something I haven't discovered yet. Unfortunately, the New York doctor made the same recommendation-steroid use. But this time, Ethan was worse because he had an infection. He needed to be put on antibiotics. I must admit I learned from this doctor that scooping out cream from a jar can be unsanitary and was probably what caused the infection. Squeeze bottles are more hygienic and can prevent contamination. But as far as curing Ethan of the eczema or finding out its cause, we were out of luck. I did not want to mask Ethan's eczema with the glossy coat of clear skin that steroids provide. I wanted Ethan to have healthy, normal skin.

We were back to using steroids- but only sporadically because I just didn't feel comfortable with them. Fortunately, the sporadic use of steroids along with various over the counter creams appeared to keep the eczema at bay. Also, everything in life is relative. Our base level for healthy skin was no longer clear, beautiful baby skin. Living with Ethan made us think that clear baby skin was as fake as the bodies of Hollywood celebrities. When Ethan would have a few good days, to us, his less than perfect skin looked liked peaches and cream.

Ethan was born in February. Springtime was tough but summer was worse. To keep him from scratching his body, which only aggravated his skin, Ethan spent his time in long shirts, and long pants tucked into his socks to prevent him from touching his own skin. Though everything he wore was cotton, in order to minimize irritation, his clothing was still too hot to spend much time outside. Still, I took him to the pool. I was not sure whether going to the pool was good or bad for him. Various dermatologists told me that chlorine would irritate his eczema. But several friends told me that the chlorine and sun do wonders to temporarily relieve their eczema. So, I did a little of both. We went to the pool every now and then. The chlorine seemed to help him a little, but the trips to the pool were worth it for another reason.

I enjoy chatting. I am not shy about striking up conversations with complete strangers. As I spoke to another mother sitting at the snack bar by the pool about Ethan's eczema, I learned something invaluable. She begged me not to put steroids on Ethan's skin. She said, "I followed everything the doctor recommended for my child's eczema, and it cleared his skin, but his skin is paper thin now that he is older. We have all kinds of problems now. Whatever you do, don't use the steroid regularly. Do anything but."

The intensity of her voice and her concern remained with me. The next time I was at the pediatrician, I asked whether thin skin was a side effect of steroid use. The response: "Of course, with long term use. But it is worth it. What else are you going to do?"

I understand doctors' bias for medicine. They are trained to prescribe medicine and often it works. But patients are rarely told of side effects. If we don't read the fine print in the several pages of small writing that comes with the box of medicine, then we would never know. Now, by profession, I am an attorney and I love to read. But rarely do I read microscopic fine print that comes with prescription medicine. Like most people, I just hope the medicine will work and don't focus on the possible side effects.

It is the doctor's responsibility to inform us but they at times do not. There are probably several reasons for this. One, low insurance reimbursements for office visits have forced doctors to see more patients in a smaller amount of time in order for them to have profitable practices. There is simply not enough time for doctors to educate their patients. Second, drug companies work hard describing to doctors the benefits of their medicines and in the process minimizing the relevance of side effects. Third, some doctors I have encountered think they have no choice but to prescribe a medicine, despite its side effects, as the only way to help a patient. Either they view the benefits to outweigh the potential side effects or they simply do not know of an alternative. Fourth, some doctors are concerned with the nocebo effect - patients causing harmful side effects simply by the suggestion that they may exist (the placebo effect in reverse). It therefore becomes our job to double check what doctors tell and give us.

When he was around seven months old, Ethan had an acute allergic reaction. I was at a swimming birthday party with all the kids. My older children were playing in the pool as I was enjoying the company and spread. They had chumus, a chickpea and sesame mixture, which is one of my favorite foods, and I ate it all afternoon. Ethan was in my arms, watching as I ate. At one point, I put a very small amount on my finger to give him a taste. I put my finger in his mouth and before I knew it, one side of his face blew up and one of his eyes swelled shut. I had never seen anything like it and did not know what to do. It also happened to be rush hour with bumper-to-bumper traffic right outside the neighborhood. Attempting to drive to the doctor would be useless; I had no idea when I would get there. I called the pediatrician, who explained that it was probably an allergic reaction and to give him Benadryl.

Thankfully, the medicine started to work quickly. By the time my husband got to the pool, he was joking that Ethan looked like Rocky after fighting Apollo Creed. Though I was pained inside, I laughed along. Somehow, I hoped my laughter would make it better. After all, he did end up okay.

In time, Ethan developed an airborne allergy to chumus. He would have an intense hive reaction that could spread throughout his entire body if we did not distance him from chumus fast enough. Through the process of elimination of ingredients, we determined that it was probably the sesame to which he was allergic. Our family and friends happen to use sesame a lot. This presented challenges when socializing, as we often turned down invitations if there was a chance that chumus would be served. (By the way, when we eventually went to an allergist, a well-known and experienced doctor, he only believed me through my repeated insistence, as he had never heard of anyone having an airborne allergy to sesame.)

It was apparent to most who saw Ethan that the redness and cuts on his face were not just newborn scratches and rosiness. Advice poured in from all around. People in the supermarket line would comment. People in synagogue would comment. My friends would comment. My family would comment. Fortunately, I am not one to take offense to this sort of thing. I actually appreciate it and believe that people's advice comes from kindness and is not an indictment on my parenting.

And so, through the kind advice of others, I found myself in an allergist's office. My doctor had been insistent that breastfed babies do not suffer from allergies; I wanted to believe him despite my experience, and had not gone to an allergist before.

I traveled to Philadelphia to see this allergist. The waiting room was packed with children of all ages. Ethan was the only infant in the room. After waiting for an hour, we finally met the allergist. He was a young doctor but like every other doctor, he owned his space and had a grand sense of command. Do they teach this in medical school? He was also filled with information that I did not know and was able to clearly relay to me some basic facts. He explained that allergy testing under the age of one was not particularly reliable. Often babies will have false positives in response to allergens to which they have no problem. But given that Ethan had such severe eczema, it was likely that he was allergic to some foods.

He gave a skin test to Ethan. This entails pricking the skin with a needle that has a bit of the potential allergen. If the skin becomes inflamed, it signifies an allergy. Ethan's results were suspect due to his overly sensitive and irritated skin. Ethan was initially diagnosed as possibly being allergic to dairy, wheat and nuts. The doctor explained to me that this test was not necessarily reliable, but since it was all we had to go on, it didn't hurt to try keeping those foods out of his system. Since I was still nursing, this meant that I had to exclude dairy, wheat and nuts from my diet. That meant that I couldn't even eat the basics like bread, pizza, peanut butter and ice cream (yes, I consider ice cream a basic). The allergist explained that even though I was nursing and the baby was not directly consuming the food I ate, in some very sensitive children what the mother eats affects the child.

I was starting to learn something very interesting. I was surprised that my pediatrician did not know the information that the allergist just explained to me. The pediatrician believed that there would be no allergy link to eczema for such a small baby who was also breastfed but the allergist explained that breastfeeding is not a guarantee that a baby will not have allergic responses. It seems that doctors are highly specialized. They sometimes don't know things outside their own areas of practice. This didn't make my pediatrician a bad doctor. In fact, I really like my pediatrician and recommend the practice to my friends. But at that moment in the allergist's office, I realized that helping Ethan should ideally be a partnership amongst me and all of his doctors, each of whom has important knowledge to impart. The allergist instructed me not to bathe Ethan too often as water has a drying effect on the skin. A number of years later I received the opposite advice from another allergist.

I left the allergist's office feeling much better. Helplessness and hopelessness are two of the worst feelings a person can have. This doctor armed me with something I could do for Ethan and for that I was grateful.

And so, I practically stopped eating. By the time Ethan was one, I had lost significant weight. For all my efforts, Ethan was better but not healed and I was almost skin and bones. I stopped nursing when Ethan turned one. I did my best to nurse as long as I could because I didn't know what Ethan would be able to eat once I stopped nursing, and I wanted to give him as much as I could for as long as I could. But the toll it was taking on my body was too much. Believe it or not just one year after the birth of a baby, after I stopped nursing, I was working on gaining weight, not losing it. Even my general doctor was concerned. Ironically, most people who saw me praised how great l looked. I received a lot of comments from women about how lucky I was and how jealous they were. The weight loss raised no warning flag in the eyes of those who viewed me with envy.

There were two main reasons I stopped nursing. One was that I was starving. I am not much of a meat eater- it does not sit well in my stomach. Not eating dairy and nuts significantly cut into my calorie intake. The second reason was that my own eczema was so severe that I had to take oral steroids to calm my skin. The doctor did not want me to take steroids while I was nursing, as they would pass through to my milk to Ethan.

I have summed up Ethan's first year quickly, but in reality it was an eternity. I had a baby who rarely slept and was uncomfortable. To exacerbate the situation, we could not even let him cry himself to sleep. Any period of excess crying (that would be anything over ten seconds) would irritate his skin, turn it red and start him scratching. The second he would start crying at night, I would have to jump out of bed and pick him up. Most nights he slept in our bed, as it was the only way he could achieve any comfort. I would be up on some level the entire night holding his hands to prevent him from scratching his body and kissing him to soothe him. By the time he reached a year, Ethan knew how to pull away his clothing to directly scratch his skin. If he could get to his skin, he would tear at it. My husband and I did not sleep through the night until he was nearly three years old.

I think that one of the main reasons that I could handle Ethan in his first few years was that I also suffered from eczema during this time. I often tore at my own skin to the point of bleeding and had to put on topical steroids and antibiotics to calm the inflammation. It was a fairly common occurrence for me to break down crying as I tried not to scratch my own skin (and then rip at it viciously.) I was able to tolerate the pain by reasoning that at least I could relate to my child.

The week Ethan turned one I made an appointment with one of the top dermatologists in New Jersey for both myself and Ethan. Again, there was the obligatory twenty minute wait before the appointment. This doctor was ancient. He did not have a single hair left on his head. He looked like he had shrunk a few inches due to the years he'd been around. But he stood straight and proud and was still clearly on top of his profession. He was worldly and began the appointment first by sharing with me some of the day's news. After the examination, it was evident that this time Ethan's skin was exceptionally overrun with eczema. He spoke clearly and slowly and persuaded me to try one week's worth of oral steroids on Ethan in an effort to snap his body out of its vicious cycle. The theory was that sometimes eczema just propels itself by the simple fact that the skin is irritated. If the skin had a chance to heal completely, maybe the eczema would not come back. I also started a round of oral steroids for my eczema.

That same week, in mid-February, my husband and I went to Florida. At the end of Ethan's first year, we were spent. Between caring for the other children, dealing with an unhappy baby and being in constant physical agony myself, there was no room for tending to our relationship. I was exhausted. My husband was in better physical shape but also drained. He works long hours in a stressful profession and is an involved father. As I spent more time tending to Ethan, he would come home and have to put the other children to sleep without my help. By the time he would sit down to eat, it would be late at night. Then as soon as we lay our heads down, a crying baby would force us to get out of bed. We typically got maybe a few hours of broken sleep per night.

Going to Florida was wondrous. First, let's give the drugs credit. I was on steroids for my eczema and my skin had that glossy steroid feeling that miraculously allowed me to be comfortable in my own skin. Second, the beach and water were beautiful. For the first time in two years I was able to immerse myself in water without breaking out in hives. The pool and ocean waters were wonderfully warm. And of course third, my husband and I were alone. We rented a convertible, put the top down, took in the breeze and just enjoyed being together.

When we returned, an amazing surprise awaited us. Ethan looked absolutely beautiful. The steroid had worked its wonders on him. His skin was baby soft. He had beautiful chubby cheeks. He was smiling. And so were we. Unfortunately, it did not last.

Traditional Medicine: Allergists And Nutritionists

After Ethan's first year, I had a constant stream of appointments with a new allergist. I live near a prominent children's hospital with an excellent international reputation (PHIR), which my pediatrician strongly recommended, I went to an allergist there. Allergy testing is considered significantly more accurate after age one.

The testing on Ethan began. Over the course of about a year, through numerous doctors appointments, blood tests, and scratch tests, we came up with a list of foods to which Ethan was allergic: chicken, beef, lamb, milk, eggs, fish, soy, nuts -I was to keep him away from all dairy, all meats, all nuts, all beans, all fish (except tuna, which I could give only a small amount once a week- for some reason he was okay with that). This list of foods also came with stern warnings from the allergist:

"Now, you want to make sure that he does not have any of these foods. The key is to keep him away from them. The less exposure he has to these foods, the more likely he is to outgrow the allergy sooner." He gave me this information by speaking methodically and clearly, in a voice that sounded three octaves lower than his normal voice, and by looking straight into my eyes, making sure I was paying attention.

Having other children, I thought that this was impossible. "I can try my best, but what you say is impossible. Ethan could easily eat a cracker with eggs, milk, soy or nuts that belongs to one of my other kids. And dairy is in everything. I am not sure I can do this one hundred percent." I responded with concern.

"Well, then do your best. It will just mean that he will outgrow the allergy later. But, you should also know that you never know what kind of reaction he will have each time he is exposed to an allergen.

You know, as he grows, instead of eczema and hives his allergic reactions will be asthmatic. This is just the pattern of allergic reactions. We don't know why this happens. We just know that it does. He might react with hives one time but then stop breathing the next." He said this both mater-of-factly and with urgency, basically saying, "Hey, get with it lady, your kid can't get near anything he is allergic to or he'll die." I am condensing several repeated conversations, which occurred over the course of testing Ethan for allergies, each with the same intent.

Every time I was given this warning, I would listen, comprehend but never accept. I did not want to live life gripped by the terror of sudden death. I did not want to subject Ethan to such a life either. "Well, I'll do my best. But it is impossible to keep him away from it all the time. He is an active baby living in a house full of kids."

Then, at one visit, my doctor says something that really shocked me. He looked up at me and speaking as if to a friend just gave me a compliment. "You have a great attitude. I can't tell you how many times I've told mothers to see a psychologist to keep their concern in perspective. Now, let's go over what you should have with you in case he has an allergic reaction."

His words took me by surprise because of the gravity of the message that he had expressed to me several times: "God forbid your kid could die." He even gave me articles supporting what he said and the importance of keeping Ethan away from the foods to which he is allergic. But then, he praised me for realizing that I could not control everything. I was shocked. I never expected this from the doctor who always set forth the worst case possibilities of an allergic reaction. Had I focused on the gravity of Ethan's allergies, I'm sure I'd be at a psychologist also. Clearly, if he was sending so many mothers to see psychologists, there was a communication gap between this doctor and his patients.

Our lives are not entirely in our hands. We can only do our best. I have a friend whose child fell from only one step and broke her neck. How can we possibly protect ourselves from everything? Ethan's list of allergies is simply too long. I can't protect him from all things all the time. What a blessing that he does not have only one allergy. I may have fallen prey to thinking that I could control his environment. I see parents who deal with a few allergies and put themselves, their children, community, and schools under such stress that their children lose a sense of normalcy.

I once had a child with a peanut allergy come to my home. His allergy was not by contact or airborne. He would have a problem only if he ingested peanut product. After lunch, he found a little brown speck on the counter. He picked it up and showed me on his finger.

"What is this?" He asked inquisitively.

"It's peanut butter." I responded. But before, I got the full words out, he completely freaked out.

He held his finger far from his body yelling in hysteria, "I'm allergic. I'm allergic. I'm allergic to peanut butter."

I asked calmly, "Did you eat any of it?" That would have concerned me. I am careful to keep the peanut butter off the table.

He replied in panic, "No." And he continued to scream, "I'm allergic to peanut butter."

I asked him again, calmly, knowing the answer, if he was contact or airborne allergic to peanut butter. Each time he yelled out repeatedly "No. No. No."

Looking straight in his eyes, I said firmly and clearly, "Okay, let's wash your hands. Here, let me put the water on for you."

He suddenly froze, looked at me, stopped yelling, washed his hands and went off to play.

I never want Ethan to be terrorized like that. All we can control in life is our approach to it. I do not want him to be a victim.

This approach has served Ethan well. Around when Ethan was four years old, he had one of his first allergic reactions that required him to use an inhaler. My mother, who was watching him at the time, was afraid to unnecessarily give him the medicine, panicked at watching her grandson having some trouble breathing and became too flustered to give him his inhaler. She called my husband, who recounts the following conversation he had with Ethan after speaking with my mom.

"Ethan, are you having a reaction?" asked my husband.

"Yeah, I just need the medicine but grandma doesn't know what to do. She won't let me do it myself without talking to you first." He replied in frustration.

"Well, go ahead and use it now. Grandma is okay with it."

"Thanks dad. I just need the inhaler that's all."

Had Ethan panicked, an easily remedied situation could have spiraled out of control landing Ethan in the emergency room. An individual in the middle of an asthma attack needs to be as calm as possible, while securing needed medicine. Panic further restricts the airways making any asthma attack more severe. Allergic fear cannot run a person's life. A person must run his own life.

Our visits to the allergist helped make sense out of some of Ethan's reactions. Ethan we learned was allergic to eggs. I noticed that Ethan's skin would become worse when I cooked eggs at home; he would always begin scratching. The allergist didn't believe me. He didn't know that anyone could have an airborne allergy to eggs. But I knew Ethan had one. I stopped cooking eggs at home with Ethan around.

One time I gave him some cereal out of a bag that also had some nuts in it. Ethan broke out in hives. We learned that he was contact allergic to nuts. When one of my children had peanut butter and then licked Ethan's face (don't ask), I had a major allergic reaction to contend with. Within moments, both his breathing and his skin were affected.

There were even some stores that I could not go into. We didn't know what he was reacting to in these stores. Home Depot was out of the question- too much dust and chemical smells. We just knew that he would break out in hives or have trouble breathing if he was there too long.

Now, let me tell you a story. Sometime around when Ethan was two, a Rabbi moved to our town. His mission was to teach Judaism to less religious Jews. We fell into this category. The Rabbi invited us and a few other families to a mountain get away one Shabbat. Shabbat in the Jewish religion is a twenty-five hour period starting each Friday evening and ending Saturday night and is filled with meals, prayers and rituals. We went to spend the weekend in the mountains to celebrate Shabbat. I say mountains but we weren't in tents camping out. Up in these mountains, there were some beautifully furnished condos with high ceilings and wide windows to view the beautiful scenery. The company was great too. We studied with the Rabbi and the children played with each other.

On a periodic check of the kids, I noticed that Ethan's cheeks were red and he was having difficulty breathing. As I try to do in these times, I sat him on my lap and calmly spoke to him. I learned that he had been crawling around on the floor eating spilled Cheerios. Cheerios he could eat. But these were Honey-Nut Cheerios. Ethan was severely allergic to nuts. Fresh air and Benadryl did him no good. And we had forgotten to bring a nebulizer, a machine that administers inhaled steroids and allows him to breathe in the event of an allergic reaction. Don't ask me why. We were deep in the mountains and had no idea where the nearest hospital was. Ethan was getting worse and having greater difficulty breathing with each passing minute. We were certainly not getting parent of the year awards.

Do you believe in God or is everything a coincidence? The Rabbi's wife happened to have a nebulizer and the medicine that Ethan required. Her child had a cold several months before that necessitated a nebulizer and for some reason in packing for this trip she brought it with her. Let me make this absolutely clear. Her child was not sick at the time. Her child never used a nebulizer before his sickness or after. She just randomly had a feeling she might need it. Well, we used the medicine and Ethan began to breathe comfortably again. Life and death are not in our hands. We do not have absolute control.

Though we did our best, Ethan's diet was a challenge. He was below the growth chart. It could be that he was naturally small or that his diet was hindering his development. I began appointments with several nutritionists at PHIR.

I don't know why but all the nutritionists at PHIR were women, each covering for the other as one of them would go out on maternity leave. It was easy to relate to them since as women and mothers we were in the same stage of life. They all recommended a hypoallergenic dietary supplement to ensure that Ethan's nutritional requirements be met. I was to make sure that Ethan had a certain amount of this formula each day. It was complete and non-allergic. What a dream. They also gave me several lists of foods that I could purchase that were, egg, dairy and soy free. The lists consisted of various cookies, cereals, crackers and other processed foods. I explained to several nutritionists that my children eat mostly fruits and vegetables and that I cooked mostly from scratch, avoiding processed and junk foods. They insisted the lists would be helpful.

Whenever I left the nutritionist's office, I always felt great. I thought they had knowledge that the doctors lacked. I thought they could best evaluate Ethan's diet. I thought they provided me with such a wonderful alternative- a complete formula. When I would leave that office, I thought my child had a better diet with his formula than most kids. And it was so easy. Just pop open the box or just mix in the powder with juice and his meal was served. No allergic reaction.

My mother, on the other hand, disagreed. Fortunately for us, as I mentioned before my mom loves nutrition and reads about it constantly (a hobby that has been of great service to us). My mother did not like Ethan's diet. My mother knows food. She is on the cutting edge of all information about nutrition. Her understanding is that food fuels the body. What goes into our body determines how our body reacts. What Ethan was given was not acceptable to her. There was no natural fat in his diet. There was no real protein. How could a child grow up healthy on a processed, chemical formula? She insisted that people are meant to eat food not formula. This argument appealed to my common sense.

Through her insistence, we became creative with Ethan's food. Since he seemed okay with olive oil and flax seed oil, we poured it on all his food- primarily vegetables, potatoes, rice and fruits. A friend, who studied nutrition in Spain, introduced me to quinoa and wild rice, both of which are high in protein. She suggested we try coconut and avocado both high in fat, the latter a very complete food. She also suggested that we give him his tuna in oil, not water, again, for greater fat. The thought had never occurred to me. Fat is very important for young children. It provides calories and is necessary for brain development.

What absolutely infuriated me was that the several nutritionists whom I saw at PHIR suggested none of this. It turned out that Ethan was allergic to both coconut and avocado but he began to eat much quinoa and wild rice, both good sources of protein. My mother encouraged me to begin experimenting with various beans. As it turns out, he was not allergic to all beans but most. We had to test each type of bean separately.

I began to question doctors more intently. I learned that many doctors think in terms of statistics. Their medical training, focused on speed and efficiency, sacrifices the extra time required to evaluate each individual. And insurance companies strongly encourage a set systematic analysis of patients. This emphasis on an evidence based medical analysis steers doctors away from creative thinking and toward rote analysis of patients. Parents as advocates for their one patient have far more time and vested interest than doctors, who are responsible for many, to search for treatment and truly understand how an illness presents itself in their child. As a result, it is often up to the patient or parent to be the diagnostician and share with doctors what they discover. Though the allergist and nutritionists were well aware of the problems of providing appropriate nutrition to a child with such a restrictive diet, no one spent time looking at his file with an eye toward expanding his diet. It was only through my questioning that Ethan's diet began to expand.

Experimentation was a very difficult process for me. I had to contend with an allergic reaction. If he reacted, I had to have medicine in hand. Ethan already had almost daily reactions, breaking out in hives on his face or arm. It was so often that I didn't always give him drugs to calm the reactions. I did not want him constantly medicated. I tried to distract him from scratching and keep him cool until his body recovered. Experimenting with a new food and the possibility of an even greater reaction was overwhelming. But every few weeks, I would have the courage to try.

It was so much easier to give Ethan the formula. The nutritionist insisted that it was a complete diet. Did I mention it was easy? So what if it cost money? I didn't have to make anything. It was easy and nothing about Ethan was easy. He cried. He scratched. He never slept. Just one easy thing was all I wanted. The doctor said give him the formula and he'll grow and get all he needs. I wanted to believe him completely. I gave Ethan the formula more often than I experimented on new foods. After all, the nutritionists and doctor insisted that it was complete and healthy. But at least Ethan had more variety in what he ate. That had to be healthier; it was just common sense.

Patient / Doctor Communication

- Write down your questions prior to your visit.
- Provide the doctor with a list of questions prior to your visit.
- If the doctor's answer seems complicated to you, repeat it to the doctor in your own words to make sure you understand the answer.
- If your doctor has an accent that you can't understand, do not hesitate to kindly ask the doctor to repeat what he says or ask for a nurse to assist you.
- If you have a question from an article, bring it to your appointment.
- Ask the same questions from all doctors that you see. Different doctors

and specialists may have different answers.
- Ask the nurses the same questions that you plan to ask doctors. Sometimes they may bring up additional issues or answer a question in a manner that is more understandable to you.
- With specialists, be sure to understand the boundaries of their knowledge.
- Remember not all doctors are great communicators. At times you will have to work hard to make sure that there are no misunderstandings.
- Specifically ask about potential side effects of a course of treatment. Educate yourself regarding the less common and long-term side effects as well.

Reike

Shortly after we returned from Florida, two important things happened. First, I read an article about the drug that suppressed the immune system- the one the doctor wanted me to use instead of the steroid. Research showed that the type of use the doctor recommended increases the chance of childhood cancer! Thankfully, I only used it a few times. I was greatly relieved and disturbed when I read this article. Every time I walked into my pediatrician's office- and for our family it was several times a month, the doctor would berate me for not following the prescribed drug regime for Ethan. Remember what he said? "You are needlessly making your child suffer." Reading the article was a boon to my confidence. There must be something to maternal instinct. Maybe mother does know best.

Second, pleasantly and unexpectedly, I found a mother's helper who would come to our home several hours a week to help me out. She was a single girl in her early twenties. I don't think of myself as old but there was an innocence and freshness to her that I remember having a decade earlier. This babysitter practiced reike.

"Haleh, you have to let me do reike on Ethan" she insisted in earnest.

"Reike? What is that?"

"It's energy. It's all around us. Let me help him. I'll give him more energy and help his body to function better."

While this sounded a little foreign to me, I do believe in the power of positive thinking. I wondered if that was reike.

"No. This has nothing to do with what I am thinking. There is energy all around us. Our body gives off energy. Look, I am not even going to touch him. Just let me work on him for a little while when he falls asleep." She was practically begging me.

I had to double check, "You are not going to touch him?" I asked in disbelief.

"No, please just trust me. Try it."

I agreed. What did I have to lose? She wasn't going to touch him and she wanted to give him energy. That didn't sound bad. I could sort of relate to this. Have you ever walked into a room where you could cut the tension with a knife? Well, that is energy. Maybe there was some logic to what she was saying.

After Ethan fell asleep, she went to his room. She shut the door, leaving only a crack for me to peak through. She stood above his crib. She raised and lowered her arms over his crib. Sometimes she waved her hands in circles. She walked all around the room waving her arms. Then she would come back to the crib and hold her arms above Ethan. I thought maybe she was praying. That could be good too. She did her arm waving, energy thing for a half hour!

Then she came out and told me the following:

"Listen, when he wakes up, he is going to be unusually hot to the touch. But he won't have a fever. It's because I gave him energy and it was his first time. He will be very relaxed. Don't worry about it. It will pass. By the way, I also sensed that you two are very connected. I think he needs to eat more meat. And you definitely have to put him in the bath more. He needs the water."

This all sounded a bit unusual. She could tell all that by waving her arms and standing around for a half-hour? It's pretty easy to imagine a Saturday Night Live skit on all this. But, here is the thing- everything happened as she said. He woke up - hot but without a fever, relaxed as can be. He never behaved this way. Usually he just cried. And the truth was Ethan and I had an unusual connection. If he itched, I itched. Often I woke up in the middle of the night moments before he would cry. If he had a good day, so did I. Maybe it was because we both had eczema and the same things bothered us both. But somehow it felt deeper than that. Besides, I had nursed him for a year and carried him most of the time in the carrier. How could we not be linked?

So, I bathed him more and I fed him meat. I had recently read an article that the latest studies recommend a regime of daily bathing for eczema with lots of moisturizer rather than limited bathing. So, I decided to try something new. Meat? Why not? He didn't have much protein in his diet, since he could not eat dairy.

I decided to try reike for my own eczema. If I was putting Ethan through this, I figured I should try it too. I paid for several sessions unsure whether the short nap that I had during the sessions was causing healing or if it was what she did. Each time I awoke from a session my reike babysitter gave me an update of what she felt. And each time, she astounded me with what she was picking up. Either she was an amazingly perceptive person or she truly was feeling my energy.

One time I had what I am told was an out of body experience. Stay with me for a minute. I would not have believed this possible if it didn't actually happen to me. I lay on the bed as I watched myself "travel" out of my body and visit family members and work through all kinds of issues. I wanted to cry but as I lay there, I was aware that I was in the middle of the reike session and did not want to cry in front of someone. I had this huge lump in my throat. Near the end of the session, I actually removed a huge metal ball from my heart and put my children in the empty space created. I woke to the sound of flowing water coming from a CD playing in the room.

Here is the amazing part. My reike babysitter had sensed in detail the range of emotions I had experienced during the session. And the best part: I felt as if the weight of the world had been lifted from me. That weekend, I laughed freer than I had in years. And that session was a turning point in the healing of my eczema, hives and various stomach ailments, all of which had gone unresolved for the past three years, despite visits to numerous specialists.

Ethan continued with weekly reike sessions. His skin, though not healed, was significantly and noticeably improved. But sadly our reike babysitter moved out of the area three months later. I was not able to find someone else who practiced reike and with whom I felt comfortable.

Mental Well Being

One thing that I consistently did with Ethan through those first years is what I call "laugh therapy". I read much about the importance of correct, deep breathing, which is credited with many health benefits. The body needs oxygen to survive and thrive. And if oxygen does not adequately reach the body, the body suffers. Now, I couldn't exactly teach a toddler to do breathing exercises. But I once read that laughter is therapeutic and has healing effects for two reasons: one, it brings joy, and two, it brings oxygen to the body. Alas, "laugh therapy" was born.

Throughout the day, I would take Ethan and tickle him. I would do this for about five minutes at a time. Despite his allergies, we want him to view life with joy. A positive view of life is paramount. At times my mom would take him at night to give us a break from the constant wake ups. In the ten-minute walk to her house she would carry and tickle him the entire way. Later when he developed asthma, we continued "laugh therapy" to strengthen his lungs. My husband's way of making him laugh was to tickle him while they wrestled.

Human psychology is a very important factor in body image and overall health (I've always been an armchair psychologist, as my husband puts it.) It was vital that Ethan view himself as healthy and strong. This by the way was not a concern that I developed on my own. Allergists, dermatologists and pediatricians all expressed concern over Ethan's mental well-being. Most children in his situation are not very easy to deal with. They are typically afraid to try new things, are not good eaters, and become quite rigid.

Ethan is the exact opposite. We credit this in part to the attitude we developed in him to live life with joy rather than the fear of what could harm him. It is not uncommon for him to say on his own, "Mom, you know, I am so lucky." I actually even used his eczema to help him develop this attitude. I would show him that his skin was cut up and then show him when it healed. "Wow!" I'd exclaim. "You are amazing. Your body just gets better. See how wonderful God made you." Instead of fearing an allergic reaction, he knows it is a process he can overcome.

Ethan's allergies showed me on a daily basis what little control we have in this life. Our attitudes, however, are ours to choose and I wanted Ethan's to be positive and strong.

His itching was the worst in the first two to three years of his life. During the day, I kept his hands occupied without ever mentioning his skin. Drawing attention to it would have only led to a power struggle. Had I tried to "explain" to Ethan that scratching didn't make him feel better and just hurt his skin more, I would not have gotten anywhere. He would have heard "you're not letting me do what I want to do and it feels good. I'm not listening to you." So we held hands and he was my little helper.

But too often Ethan would go to bed looking okay and then wake up in the morning cut up. He was scratching himself at night. Even though we had him in a one piece, zipped stretchy at all times, his hands were still free. At night, I could only control his hands when he slept with us, which was only three or four nights a week. I couldn't do this every night because . . . do I need to explain how desperately exhausted I was? So I came up with ways to keep his hands busy at night without him knowing it.

My daughter gave Ethan one of her baby dolls to hug and sleep with and I covered Ethan's hands with socks. It's all in the approach. On the socks, I drew faces and each night had a puppet show with him before he went to bed. Then, he kept those puppets on at night. He went to bed with a smile and perfectly content to keep his hands covered with the puppets, hugging his baby to sleep.

One day, when he was four and half, he put socks on his hands, came running to me with a big smile on his face and asked if I remembered doing puppet shows with him when he was little. He wanted me to do it again. He loved it. To be honest, at first my heart tightened as I remembered the stress of those days. But then I smiled, as I realized that on an instinctual, deep level, he views his childhood in happiness.

Now, not everything I did was discrete. Ethan was well aware of his allergies. He learned that himself fairly quickly. It was not uncommon for him to eat something and then throw up. That was partly how we discovered his fish allergy. But we focused on what he could eat, not his limitations. I educated him. As soon as he learned to talk, he asked about ingredients of foods he was offered. If we had to list what he could not eat, we always followed it with the even longer list of what he could eat. We would list each fruit and vegetable separately, every type of rice dish separately, mashed potatoes were separate from french fries. And then, as we told Ethan when he would get older, he would outgrow his allergies. Ethan understood this and would often say, "I am not going to allergy when I am big." For Ethan, this was all part of growing up. Hope is something I am not willing to take away.

The other children are wonderful with Ethan. They are aware of his allergies and are careful in sharing food with him. But at the same time, they do not handle him like a fragile child. Ethan is one of the gang. They hold no resentment towards him for the additional considerations he requires. I have been very careful not to let our lives revolve around Ethan for everyone's sake. When Ethan has an allergic reaction, I handle it like any other normal activity. In the middle of doing homework with one of the kids, I'll casually give Ethan the medicine he needs and just get back to homework. Often, I'll continue doing whatever I was doing and give him the medicine without any interruption at all. At most, unless severe, Ethan's allergic reactions are treated like a call waiting in the middle of a phone conversation.

His stash of medicine, inhaler, and epi pen, are not kept in a medicine bag. They are in "The Superman Bag." I bought his brother a Superman backpack that came with a very large pencil case, with a Superman logo. He kindly gave the pencil case to Ethan; we use it for Ethan's medicine. It is "The Superman Bag." Though Ethan is on the lower end of the growth chart, he believes he is stronger and more able than other kids his age. And since he is "Superman," he is always willing to try new things and knows he can overcome challenges.

We cannot control the hand we are dealt. We can control our attitude and actions. A child's positive attitude can keep him calm and cooperative in the midst of a crisis. A child's hope can give him strength to try new things and courage to feel comfortable despite "uniqueness". Life is a self-fulfilling prophecy. A perceived sense of good health helps to achieve health in the face of illness.

Too often patients are pigeonholed with their prognosis based only on statistical data. This can result in stamping out hope of greater wellness in patients and discouraging patients to try alternative treatments. The power of the mind and its vast importance in healing should be harnessed more effectively.

The power of mind is well documented in medicine. It is called the placebo effect. Even when patients are given a sugar pill that is said will heal their particular ailment, there is always a large percentage of those people who actually heal because they believe the "medicine" they are given will work for them. But some doctors not only do not use this power in their favor, they actually do the opposite. Doctors may be concerned with the ethical implications of not being completely honest with patients and therefore share all negative news. As parents, we can request doctors to speak with us separately, without our children. We, as parents, can then filter the positive to our children while being aware of the negative in the back of our minds.

Efforts by patients to search for a remedy for their ailments outside of the confines of traditional medicine are at times stifled. Navigating the boundaries of evidence based medicine and alternative treatments is a challenge for doctors. This may be due to a doctor's concern not to make a mistake or a doctor's concern not to support unsubstantiated miracle cures. Unfortunately, the result is that often doctors do not become partners in care for each patient's particular needs. Rather than bolster a person's natural optimism and instinct for survival, a doctor's conservative and methodical approach has the direct effect of presenting the doctor's treatment as the only panacea. It is our responsibility to maintain hope and an open mind when faced with any diagnosis. If we can partner with our doctors in this vision, that is preferred. If we cannot, persist, persist, persist, for only this will lead to greater healing.

One Last Effort: Steroids And Anti-Biotics

Having young children, one of whom had severe allergies, was a source of much stress. My in-laws and my husband thought that it was time for a family vacation. So, my in-laws offered to treat us to a family vacation in South Carolina.

As nice as the thought was, I was not interested in the fourteen-hour drive that it would take to get there. Call me crazy, but the thought of driving so many hours, in a confined car, with little children, did not sound like a vacation to me. But we made it work. We had every car game known to man and a few I made up. I had a box of food up front ready to feed any grumpy child. And each child had his own pillow and blanket.

I'll spare you our "vacation pictures" and get right to what we discovered about Ethan. Every day that week, we spent several hours hanging out in the pool. Ethan had a little floater with a cover to block the sun. The prolonged immersion in water affected Ethan's skin. In place of the usual scabs on his legs and arms, there were indentations on his skin. It clearly looked to me as if his skin was infected and the water and chlorine opened and cleaned the infection. As the week progressed, his skin looked significantly better.

Upon our return, a visit to the dermatologist confirmed what I thought and brought us to a new approach. It is not unusual for skin that has eczema to be infected. While Ethan's skin didn't appear to be infected, it probably had been. He was placed on antibiotics to heal the skin followed by a full month of oral steroids to try once again to snap his body out of the eczematic cycle. Remember, we had tried this approach before, but not in conjunction with antibiotics and not for an entire month. We were hopeful.

Well, as long as he was on the drugs, he was fine. As soon as we stopped the steroids, his eczema was back again. The drugs simply masked a problem that never went away.

Dr. Dianne

One of the gifts that we can have in our lives is to surround ourselves with good people. Our fortune was to stumble on Dr. Dianne, one of those rare individuals who go beyond the call of duty. Dr. Dianne is not a medical doctor; she is a speech therapist. But her expertise and dedication to healing makes her our "Dr. Dianne". Dr. Dianne was our daughter's speech therapist; she would actually call my daughter at home to make sure that she was doing her exercises. Often, when we went to speech, I had the other children with me.

"Haleh, Ethan has such a bad rash on his face; he is all red. Is he okay?" She asked with genuine concern.

"Yes. He has allergies and severe eczema. The doctors want me to use steroids to soothe it but I only do it when it's really bad. It won't cure it." I respond casually.

"Isn't there something they can do for him?" she'd asked softly with a sigh in her voice.

"He'll outgrow this," I state firmly.

"But maybe we can help him outgrow it more quickly or have him be more comfortable in the process," she pressed on.

Our friendship began. Weekly, after the speech session, she would inquire after Ethan. At the time, I was in the midst of going through dermatologists, allergists, pediatricians and nutritionists for their opinions.

Dr. Dianne encouraged me to seek alternative remedies. I am actually very open to alternative therapies. I have seen, first hand, home remedies from the old country that sometimes work faster than drugs. Ever try watermelon to bring down a fever? It works wonders on a kid who won't take medicine. Growing up, medicine was turned to as a last resort not a first.

There were several reasons why I had not pursued alternative treatments. First, the visits to the allergists, nutritionists, dermatologists and pediatricians, not to mention the various medical tests, kept me pretty busy. Second, I wanted to be sure that I had done everything that medicine had to offer. Despite medicine being the last resort when I was growing up, I still looked to doctors as bastions of overflowing knowledge. Aren't doctors the smartest of the bunch? They have all the answers; modern medicine is a gift. I respect doctors. I did not completely respect the "alternative" world that had not yet been tested by our medical community. And, finally, did I mention the cost? None of the alternative treatments were covered by our insurance. The first appointments and accompanied testing are rather costly.

But Dr. Dianne was insistent. She had found in her practice that no ailment can be treated in isolation. Even something as seemingly isolated as a speech problem could be a sign of other issues. For example, if a child has problems with chewing foods of different textures, it may be that the child is simply having a battle of wills with his parents. It could be that the child is sensitive or allergic to the foods being given. It could be that the child is missing the vitamins or nutrients that strengthen the jaw muscles. It could be something else entirely. Nothing is in isolation and, in Dr. Dianne's experience, speech therapy at times requires a physical work up.

During one of the speech therapy sessions, she sat me down to watch a video explaining alternative philosophy. The video explained that the human body is a complex machine. This machine works efficiently and requires all of its components to function. When the machine breaks down, rarely is there one reason for it. If a person is not functioning well, looking to medicine alone often does not deal with the source of the breakdown. Psychological, emotional, energy, nutritional, mineral, herbal, medical and physical treatments all have to be considered. This made sense to me.

As I mentioned, I had been dealing with my own physical challenges. I had gone to general doctors, allergists, endocrinologists, gastroenterologists, dermatologists, and physical therapists in search of a cure for my eczema and stomach problems. The diagnosis: "Stress. Here are some drugs to calm your nerves." I never took the drugs. Why mask stress? I had to change my life. What I had discovered was that reike, yoga, exercise, friends, and taking time out for myself went a long way. And as I would discover a few years later, thanks to my mom, a vegetable juice diet is what I ultimately needed to return me to complete health.

The video that Dr. Dianne showed me was something I understood and with which I grew up but had not followed with my son. Over the course of several months, Dr. Dianne convinced me to go see my first alternative doctor. I agreed. Avoiding most foods, letting Ethan live on formula, and constantly giving him steroids was not acceptable.

I wanted Ethan healed, not limited. What we discovered changed Ethan's life.

The Healing Potential

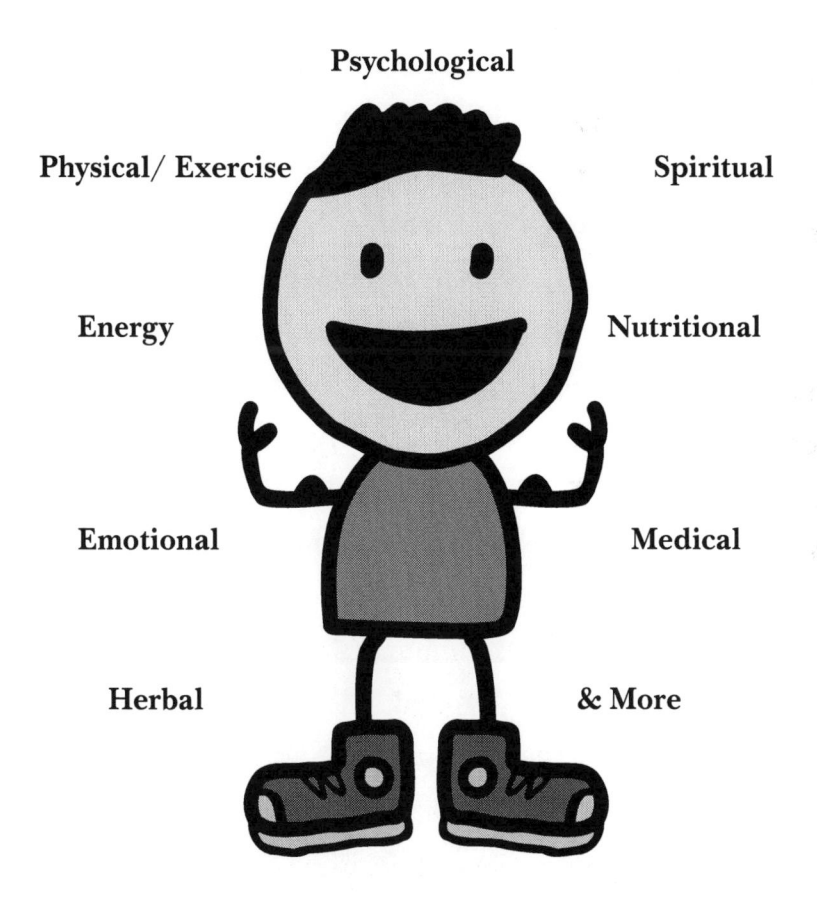

Psychological

Physical/ Exercise

Spiritual

Energy

Nutritional

Emotional

Medical

Herbal

& More

Alternative Doctors

The doctor to whom Dr. Dianne introduced me had a medical degree, but after years in traditional medicine had decided to focus his practice on alternative healing. What is alternative healing? It is one way to define any remedy that is not medically tested and authorized by United States' standards. I respect the scientific approach but we have much to learn from other cultures.

I drove over an hour away with Ethan to this doctor's office. It looked like any other from the outside, part of a complex of office buildings. Inside was unremarkable, a typical waiting area and receptionist with the standard minimum twenty minute wait for the doctor. While I waited, I noticed an area where some older patients were receiving an intravenous drip of some sort. It was upsetting to see this. I thought how desperate must I be to bring my child here and what exactly was going on? I was a little scared- there was no way I would agree to something like this for Ethan.

When we went back to the doctor's office, what I noticed first was the massive bookcase that took over the entire wall behind the doctor's desk. This was no ordinary examining room. Of course the standard bed, blood pressure gauge, sink and various diplomas on the wall also occupied the room.

The doctor had a disarming manner about him as he explained his disenchantment with traditional medicine. After years of questioning and resistance from fellow doctors to non-familiar approaches, he had set out on his own to practice "alternative medicine." He explained that many of his colleagues did not agree with what he had learned through years of experience and study of healing. Conformity and standard treatment provide traditional doctors with the hallmark of consistency that help prove a particular treatment to be useful. In the "alternative world" we'd have to experiment with Ethan together. I peppered him with questions and through several visits shared with him the skepticism I received from other doctors. Each time he answered my questions and directed me to additional sources for further clarification or support.

Through rounds of tests we discovered that in addition to Ethan's allergies he has "sensitivities" to another twenty foods. These "sensitivities" could cause minor irritations in his gut or even allergic like symptoms. The concept of food sensitivities is not supported by the traditional medical community, which only focuses on allergic responses to food proteins. Ethan had been tested for and was not considered allergic to some of the foods to which he was sensitive. (Ethan's allergist did not believe that there was any credible medical support for food sensitivities.) Now we had another whole group of foods to avoid. I finally had an explanation for why his skin was always red after the oatmeal baths that were suppose to calm his skin. He was sensitive to oats.

The doctor also prescribed probiotics and fish oil. As a result of all the antibiotics that Ethan had taken, his gut lacked sufficient "good" bacteria. Antibiotics, in doing their work, also kill good bacteria that exist and are necessary in our body. Good bacteria help in food digestion. Probiotics help to replace some of the naturally occurring bacteria that exist in the body. Had Ethan not been allergic to yogurt, he may have been able to replenish what he needed that way (yogurt is filled with natural, good bacteria). With proper bacteria levels, Ethan could digest and use the nutrients in the food he ate more efficiently. The fish oil that the doctor prescribed ensured that Ethan would receive fat in his diet that was also largely missing. Ethan was primarily eating only fruits and vegetables at this time. Additionally, the doctor was hopeful that the fish oil would also heal his skin.

This alternative doctor echoed what the allergist and pediatrician said about Ethan. They were all impressed to see how well he was doing developmentally. He did not have ADD or the typical physical or speech developmental delays associated with children with such severe allergies. In fact, he was very focused, energetic, well spoken and advanced for his age. Unlike my allergist and pediatrician who chalked it up to luck, he had an explanation. Ethan's diet to date, which he owed to the advice of my mother and my friend who had her nutrition degree from Spain, was varied. Though he could not eat traditional sources of protein and fat, he was eating quinoa, wild rice, olive oil and many fruits and vegetables. Ethan did not have as many nutritional deficiencies as most kids in his situation. He was not developmentally delayed.

Additionally, the doctor told me to stop giving Ethan formula. At this point, though Ethan ate other foods to provide a complete diet, the formula was still a large part of Ethan's caloric intake. Although it was supposed to be hypo-allergenic, the first few ingredients of the formula were items to which Ethan was sensitive.

I started to experiment and took the formula away for a couple of days. He was drinking the formula in the form of a juice box, which he loved. What I noticed was stunning. Within a day, a sore he had next to his lip disappeared. Within two days, his overall skin looked better. I thought maybe it was coincidence. I gave him the "juice" box again. The sore returned to his lip. I stopped giving him the "juice". The sore disappeared. I tested this several times with the same results each time. I couldn't believe it. Clearly Ethan was showing a reaction to this hypo-allergenic formula that the nutritionists and allergist had recommended and repeatedly told me would illicit no allergic reaction. I called the formula company, which confirmed that a very small percentage of kids do have a reaction to the juice box but not their powder formula. From that day, I stopped giving him formula entirely. I just had enough. Even if the powder version of the formula was safe, I didn't trust the process anymore and I just wanted my child to eat real food.

Almost overnight, Ethan was able to wear normal clothes. He was no longer wearing the one piece zipped up pajama. He was no longer scratching his body uncontrollably. He began to lose his airborne allergies to egg and sesame.

Within weeks he had a growth spurt. His head finally passed the kitchen counter. This was significant. Until this point, Ethan had not been on the growth charts. We had even taken an x-ray to ensure that there were no growth issues.

Within a month, the quality of Ethan's skin was better than it had ever been. None of the topical creams we tried came close to what the fish oil was repairing internally.

Shortly after, Dr. Dianne referred me to a nutritionist. From the beginning I was impressed with this woman. She was kind enough to talk to me over the phone and not demand that I go to her office which was several states away. Since she had a relationship with Dr. Diane, they worked together to help Ethan. Dr. Diane listened in on many phone conversations to help clarify and explain what I could not.

Like the PHIR nutritionists, this nutritionist requested a list of all the foods that Ethan ate over the course of three days. Unlike the other nutritionists, who had nothing to tell me until the list of foods was inputted into a computer, she immediately located Ethan's deficiencies. She stated exactly what the other nutritionists' computer print out had and then continued with a discussion of how digestion works in the body.

She explained that Ethan's gut was in a state of disrepair. Constant allergic reactions damaged his gut. This resulted in his body's inability to absorb food properly. Also, a damaged gut results in leakage of food proteins into the blood stream, which elicits allergic reactions. What we needed to do was to heal his gut, while simultaneously aiding his digestion until he was fully healed. We began to give Ethan calcium and magnesium supplements, which both addressed a deficiency in his diet and also helped him heal internally. Additionally, we gave him enzymes to help him with digestion.

Though this all made sense to me, I checked with Ethan's pediatrician. Not surprisingly, he didn't agree with this new plan. According to him, the nutritionist didn't understand the entirety of the digestion process. I didn't have a medical degree to even begin to determine who was right. But to be safe, I confirmed with the pediatrician that the digestive enzymes wouldn't cause him any harm. And then, I went along and tried it. I was thankful that my doctor did not outright forbid me from trying the enzymes. Good doctors struggle with the point at which it is safe to support patients to try these alternative methods. Because they are not extensively tested, they can pose harm.

The experimentation began once again. Lentil was a bean to which Ethan had tested sensitive but not allergic. But every time he ate lentils, he would break out in hives. Despite this, the allergist insisted that Ethan could eat lentils without a problem. I noticed that when I gave Ethan the enzyme he was able to eat lentils without breaking out in hives. When I did not give him the enzyme, he would break out in hives. The enzyme was definitely doing something. I also noticed that Ethan no longer had extremely soft stools. His stools became normal. This, according to the nutritionist, signaled that Ethan's body was absorbing more nutrients from the food he ate.

On a routine visit to the allergist, the doctor was surprised at how well Ethan was doing. Although he believed that Ethan would naturally outgrow his eczema and then have asthma, he was still impressed. He had never seen a child improve so dramatically. When I explained the alternative methods I used, the doctor shrugged his shoulders and said, "I don't believe that stuff. There is no support for it. But if you want to keep doing it, go ahead." I suggested he share my experience with other patients. I asked him to contact Ethan's alternative doctors. He shook his head at both suggestions. He just didn't accept what I was doing, despite the evidence in front of him of Ethan's remarkable improvement.

Not all doctors are the same. Some are more receptive to alternative methods than others. One doctor said to me, "You know, the problem is that most of these alternative methods just have not been scientifically tested in America. They come from other countries and we are just not familiar with them. There aren't enough studies supporting whether they work. Of course, it's possible that something I don't know about works. Just keep me in the loop as you try new things, especially if you start taking herbal supplements. Some of those are potent and may not mix well with some medications." What's the difference? It's in the approach. One discourages and the other encourages patients to seek out remedies and help themselves.

At this point, Ethan was on the verge of having his tonsils taken out. He snored through the night and a sleep study revealed that he had severe sleep apnea. Through the years his allergies had caused him to have enlarged tonsils, which were causing him some difficulty at night. But only days before the scheduled tonsillectomy, we cancelled. Ethan was no longer snoring at night. He was no longer waking up. At almost three and half he was finally sleeping through the night.

Our new nutritionist explained that a decrease in gut irritation could be responsible for the change. There was less mucus buildup in the gut that might have been backing up into the lungs. Also, his body was simply working better, resting and healing. I spoke with a pulmonologist about this theory. He wasn't sure he agreed with it, but he did not discount it either. As a doctor from outside our medical establishment, he was a believer in the effect of nutrition on overall health.

Just as the allergist predicted, Ethan outgrew his eczema only to become asthmatic. Still, we impressed the allergist with Ethan's speedy recovery with eczema and Ethan impressed everyone with his normal mental and physical development despite his severe allergies. We are hopeful to do the same with his asthma. He is active and well adjusted. His sensitivities to food allergens are reduced and continue to decrease. Instead of worse reactions with repeated exposure, Ethan has less severe reactions. We still visit the emergency room on occasion, but, thankfully, he recovers faster than his doctors predict. Ethan is not a victim. He has a very strong self-image, is fearless, and has a zest for life.

We still go to the allergist. We still carry the Superman bag. We still look to alternative treatments. Right now Ethan is eating goji berries, which some claim have healing benefits. We are also working on guided imagery to stay calm and help Ethan recover from minor allergic reactions on his own without medicine. What we have learned is that alternative methods must supplement and sometimes supplant western traditional medicine. It is the whole package, addressing Ethan's nutritional, psychological, emotional, spiritual, energy and physical needs that lead to our success with our healthy, feisty Ethan.

Navigating Possibilities

- Be receptive to treatment options beyond what you know.
- What doesn't work today may work tomorrow.
- Be open to trying alternative methods at different times during an illness.
- When searching the web, always check the source of information. Not all sites are equally reputable.
- Ask for references when considering an alternative healer.
- There are medical doctors who also practice "alternative medicine". Be sure to confirm their credentials.
- Some insurance companies cover what was once considered alternative. Visits to some healers and even

nutritional supplements may be covered by your insurance.
- When using herbal remedies and other supplements, be sure to share this information with your medical doctor and pharmacists. Certain combinations of medicine and herbal remedies or supplements may be dangerous.
- Ask your doctor to be a partner with you in your search for various treatments.

ALEX

Three and a half years have passed since Ethan was born and I am again in labor. I tried the prayer I used when delivering Ethan. I often turned to it in times of difficulty to give me strength. It reminded me that no matter what I was facing I would be okay. I tried the prayer again.

I am with God, God is with me;
I have the power and strength of God.
I am with God, God is with me;
I have the power and strength of God.
I am with God, God is with me;
I have the power and strength of God.

It wasn't working. I tried again.

I am with God, God is with me;
I have the power and strength of God.

I am with God, God is with me;
I have the power and strength of God.

And again.

I am with God, God is with me;
I have the power and strength of God.

I finally gave up and begged for an epidural. The faster they could get it to me the better. I just couldn't take the pain anymore. When the anesthesiologist came to prep me, I broke down in tears.

As I cried, I asked the nurses for assurance. "Will my kids be healthy? Can I raise them all to be happy, emotionally stable people? How can I possibly do it? I have to be there for them around the clock, so please, please, please don't mess up. Hey, Doc, you seem like such a nice person, don't paralyze me or anything. Promise? Please, promise that I can do this. Will my kids all be okay?"

We all have these thoughts of self-doubt and fear when we have a child. After all, they are normal fears - but, for me, never until now. And as my tears and fears poured out, I knew exactly why my prayer did not work this time. I did not have the same faith in my strength and abilities. It was as if I suddenly realized that I was a mother. I did not have the same faith in God. I feared tomorrow so much, that it sapped my energy to draw on God's strength when I needed it. I didn't even know I had so much fear inside of me.

Even after they gave me the epidural, I kept crying and shaking. I couldn't stop feeling the pain. They gave me such a large dose; I didn't feel my legs for quite a while after giving birth. In the past, I would get up and walk right after the delivery, even with an epidural. Now, I cried and shook even after the pain went away. I cried and shook until for some reason I started to laugh and my laughter pushed Alex into this world. Need I describe him? As you know already, like all mother's babies, he looks like an angel too.

Those two days in the "Hospital-Hotel" were amazing. As anyone with multiple kids can vouch, the forty eight hours covered by insurance is the most valuable gift a new mom can receive. For those precious hours, I took care of me. The baby stayed in my room only to nurse. It was easy and breezy and just plain fun.

Alex was born September fourth. We had to go home the morning of September sixth. This was the first day of school. My husband went to the opening assembly at eight-thirty with the children. Everything seemed to be going smoothly until he tried to leave at nine o'clock. Our new kindergartner started to cry and clung on to him and wouldn't let go. It was actually surprising since he knew the school, had been there many times with the other kids, and was a very adaptable and laid back child. But that didn't stop him from going to pieces. Finally, with the help of a few wonderful teachers, he was pried off my husband who then rushed out, Ethan in tow, to pick me and the baby up from the hospital. He had to be back to the office for a twelve o'clock lunch meeting.

My husband believes that doctors respect his time; maybe he demands it more than I do. I have lost count of the number of hours I've spent waiting for doctors. My husband was under the impression that everything would run like clock work and we would actually leave the hospital by ten-thirty as planned. I was ready when he arrived but the hospital was not.

We were waiting for some test results. After pacing the halls, tracking down doctors and eating lunch at the hospital, we finally get the results. My husband looks at the doctor impatiently and rolls his eyes in frustration; he was still hoping he could make it to his meeting in time. These routine tests were meaningless to him. The baby looked fine. That was all he needed. Except that the baby failed his newborn hearing test in one ear. We ask, what does that mean? The response: probably nothing. He probably has some fluid in his ears; we should take another test. What? If it's fluid, can't we do this later? Yes. Okay, great, we are leaving. We had no time to stick around just to be reassured that everything was okay in the end.

We were all thrilled to walk out the hospital doors. I wanted to check on my kindergartner. My husband had to get to work. Ethan was getting tired of the hospital room. And Alex, well, like any angel, he was asleep- which meant we had to get him home before he started crying uncontrollably in the car.

Week One: Welcome Home

Did I mention that five days before Alex was born, the kids flooded our basement? They left the outside hose running right by the basement window. By the time we found out, the carpet was destroyed. The paneling and underlying drywall and drop ceiling all had to be cut out to dry out the basement. Oh, and the heater broke down- it was over thirty years old. And of course my husband had to get new tires for his car.

And then the bris... Jewish boys are circumcised eight days after birth to welcome them into the tribe of Israel. We were having the bris in our home. We believe that the home should be the site of joyous occasions, so we try to celebrate in our home. But having a party in our home, eight days after the baby is born, is not easy.

The mohel is the man who performs the actual circumcision. Despite this man's experience and good credentials, I did not feel comfortable with him. After the mohel left, I took Alex to our pediatrician. Watching the doctor unwrap his bleeding penis was no fun. The doctor told me that the mohel had done a fine job. He just cut a little more skin than is necessary (my husband insists I mention that this does not affect the size . . . something about family honor). It was his method of doing the circumcision- nothing to worry about. It would heal without a problem but I had to return in two days to make sure the bleeding stopped.

Two days later was Rosh Hashana, the Jewish New Year, and one of the most important days to attend synagogue. It was already a bit much getting everyone dressed and ready. The last thing I wanted was to go back to the doctor. But go back I did. When the doctor looked, Alex was still bleeding. She wanted me to go to a urologist. None would see me. They wanted me to go to PHIR- just in case there was a problem. Great. Now, I had to involve my husband.

We arrive at PHIR just to wait and wait. Finally, we go in and a nurse wants to examine Alex first. We explained that we didn't want her to open the wound only to have it reopened by another doctor on call and then again by the urologist. And so we waited and waited until the urologist was available.

When the urologist arrived, he came with a crew: two attending doctors, the intern, the nurse, as well as some specialist. They took little ten-day old Alex and placed him on a standard hospital bed with crisp white sheets. They pulled out a very bright and large light and shined it right on his lower half. Then, they removed his diaper. Alex laid there, without saying a word, naked from the waist down with little legs kicking in the air. He was then unbandaged as six professionals and two anxious parents lean in for a closer look at the goods. The scene was comical, a sitcom moment. The results? No blood. Nothing. All healed. Little did I know he was going to repeat this pattern.

We pack him up and head home.

Week Two: Settling In

I am trying to find a routine for the kids at the start of school. There are lots of phone calls to make as I work on finding someone to repair the heater before winter starts. The basement cleaning process continues.

Week Three: Aladdin- Kids Can't Fly

My daughter has a friend over. The kids decide to play "Aladdin" with Ethan. They put him on a mattress and raise him in the air. He falls flat on his face and is bleeding profusely. Grab the baby. Grab Ethan and get moving. Emergency Room. Dental Office. Anti-biotic for the deep cuts. Dead grayed front baby teeth. No damage to adult teeth. Thank God.

Week Four:
Sukkot- Live It Up

Each year I invite all the children in each of my kids' classes to our home for the Jewish holiday of Sukkot. We always put up a succah for the holiday. A succah is a temporary outdoor hut built to remind us of the forty years Jews wondered the desert after being slaves in Egypt. I had absolutely no desire to have any guests. I just had a baby and a few very hectic weeks. But having guests is part of the holiday. Not partying in the succah is like having Christmas without the dinner. There was no way that I could not have these get togethers. So, each of my children had their individual parties, inviting all their classmates and friends. They were thrilled. I was beat.

I had a checkup for one of my kids - everything is fine. A hearing test for our nine-year old daughter was the other medical task for this week. My husband suspected that she had a hearing problem because she didn't always answer him when he called her. Sounded like a normal kid to me but better safe than sorry. She went into a sound booth for a hearing test. A sound booth is an absolutely silent room, insulated from outside noises. She put on headphones as she was asked to raise her hand to indicate from which ear she heard a particular sound. Of course, her hearing was absolutely normal- actually, it was a little better than normal. Kids ignore their parents until they call out to them at least fifty times- no less.

No matter how organized I try to be, no matter how much I try to be on top of all of the kids' activities- I can't do it all. On most nights, my husband comes home to put the kids to sleep, I am simply too tired by nighttime to do it on my own. The baby doesn't sleep at night and the days are, well, busy. I don't remember if I had a chance to shower anytime this month. Oh, maybe I did this morning - I just can't remember - was that just twelve hours ago?

Week Five: Rocking The Boat

Alex has his one-month check up. Everything is fine. Everything is always fine, right? I am not sure why I have this attitude. It is not as if I haven't seen hardship. I know many who have had to deal with cancer or other major illnesses. But I still think that everything is always fine.

My calendar says "Get Anniversary Gift". Would you believe that life has been so hectic that I am afraid of forgetting our anniversary in two weeks? Hopefully, this works.

At the end of this week, I have to recheck Alex's ear. Remember, he didn't pass his newborn hearing test. Even though I know everything is always fine, I had to get it checked. I went to the PHIR to get an ABR, a test that measures brainwaves in response to clicking sounds that are sounded in the ear. An ABR is used because newborns don't have the head control necessary to turn their heads toward a sound to show that they are hearing.

First, I have to make sure that Alex falls asleep. The room is absolutely silent to help with this- odd- our home is never silent. I wondered if for Alex noise would be more helpful. There is even a rocking chair in the room. The audiologist helps by dimming the lights in the room and bringing a pillow for me to rest my arm on as I rock him to sleep. Wow, I really like this woman and she has such a nice reassuring smile. I felt sure that this was just a nice break from my hectic schedule.

After Alex falls asleep, the audiologist places a couple of wires on his head and ears. (Two years earlier, I had to get a sleep study done for Ethan. He must have had at least twenty to thirty wires attached all over his body. So, a couple of wires attached to little Alex's head didn't upset me too much- although, I would rather see him in a cute hat.)

I watch as the audiologist types on a keyboard at first with confidence and then with a quizzical look on her face. She reaches to adjust the hearing piece, fiddles with the computer some more, but still looks puzzled. A veteran of medical testing, by now, this did not look good to me. She must have sensed my concern and kindly began to reassure me.

"Sometimes the ear plugs aren't in correctly."

"Is there a problem?" I ask.

"I'm just not getting a very good reading. Let me try something else." She says, as she begins to type again on the keyboard.

I next ask the question which I hope she answers in the positive. "Is there something wrong with the computer?"

"No, that's not it. I'm just not getting a good reading. Let me check the other ear and see what's going on."

This doesn't sound good to me. It seems that there's something wrong. I wait as patiently as I can, while she adjusts wires and keeps typing. I know that she is the professional but the more she readjusts the ear piece, the more I hope that she just has no idea what she's doing.

After three different types of hearing tests that day, the audiologist tells me that Alex has unilateral hearing loss. This meant that Alex had normal hearing in one ear but could not hear out of the other one. Now, let me tell you something about myself. I can ask a lot of questions. I peppered her with countless inquires over the next half hour. She answered with patience, knowledge and understanding.

As much as I didn't like that Alex couldn't hear out of one ear, it wasn't too upsetting. My father had lost his hearing in one ear as a child due to repeated, untreated ear infections. He had trouble locating the sound of a ringing telephone, and the TV was always too loud; other than that, my father leads a completely normal and successful life. So, the news of hearing loss in one ear was not overly upsetting. The audiologist told me that I needed to return in three weeks to confirm the results with a sedated ABR. It was standard to have a sedated ABR, but since Alex had slept so soundly throughout this test, she believed that the sedated ABR would only confirm what she discovered.

Of course I went home and straight onto the internet. I did some research and learned everything I possibly could about unilateral hearing loss. Not too bad. Speech develops normally. No hearing aid is needed. Many people have unilateral hearing loss and it goes undetected. The biggest issue is that during school years, a child with unilateral hearing loss should sit in the front row. That is because localizing sound is difficult without both ears and it is easy not to pay attention if you are not focused on the sound. Not too bad. I think we'll live.

Weeks Six - Eight: All You Need Is Your Health

These weeks pass with various doctor appointments: pediatrician, nutritionist, dentist, gynecologist and podiatrist. Preventative care takes time too. I think one blessing of a busy life is that there is no time to make a mountain out of a molehill. Time flies by with a mind of its own and with never a dull moment.

Week Nine: No Sleep For The Weary

The sedated ABR is this week. We take Alex back to confirm the diagnosis of unilateral hearing loss. Alex first had to see an ENT to ensure that his ears were clear for the test. The ENT had a business-like demeanor about him. There were many patients in the waiting room and ours was a routine visit- he just had to make sure Alex's ears were clear. His possible diagnosis of unilateral hearing loss was nothing extraordinary or eventful to this ENT.

Since Alex had to be sedated, a nurse had to be present to monitor him during the ABR. A different audiologist sees us this time. She is equally as kind and patient as the previous audiologist and ever helpful as Alex falls asleep.

My husband accompanies me on this visit. His eyes bug out when he sees all the wires and machinations involved. This time though, after adjusting and readjusting the earpiece, the results turn out worse than before. An hour and a half later, after numerous questions we walk out exhausted and dazed.

Now the diagnosis is that Alex has moderate to severe hearing loss in both ears. He needs hearing aids. We were told that his hearing loss was so significant that if he didn't get hearing aids by the time he was six months old, he risked never being able to speak normally. We now had to do a complete work-up on Alex to ensure that there was nothing else wrong with him. The tests included: EKG, eye test, MRI, blood tests as well as follow up hearing tests.

None of this was making much sense to me. Our son seemed absolutely normal. He showed no signs of not being able to hear. I'd had babies before. I felt strongly that if he could barely hear, I would know. I spent lots of time with him and often witnessed him waking up at the slightest sounds. Sometimes he slept heavily, but what baby doesn't? Also, the change in test results was curious. It was only three weeks after the previous test; yet, there was such a dramatic difference between them. Neither the audiologist nor the ENT could explain what was going on. We needed to schedule another ABR to confirm the results.

We both walked out of the appointment shell-shocked. Still, I got on the phone right away. Making the appointments took hours. Call. Get transferred. Transferred again. Wrong department. Get disconnected. Get an appointment months away. Get primary doctor to call to make it sooner. Call back. Lunch break. Transferred. Wrong department. Try again. I kid you not. This is what it takes. My days of constant phone calls were just beginning.

Did I mention that I have other children who happen not to have school for two days this week? I had playdates and kids screaming in the background as I worked the phone for Alex.

By week's end, I had scheduled Alex for an EKG. I was anxious but tried not to show it. I had no idea what an EKG was. I knew it had to do with the heart, I couldn't even begin to guess how complicated this test was going to be. A heart test? I'd never had one of those before.

But I thought to myself, what's the use of being nervous? Everything turns out for the best. Besides, if I show that I am upset, everyone else will become more upset. My motto is to play it cool. Some believe that it's better to prepare for the worst and hope for the best. I don't agree. What does that mean anyway? If you prepare for the worst, you won't even be able to accept the best when it comes along. Prepare for the best and expect the best. The worst - well, that'll turn out for the best too. What's the use of being completely stressed out? If I prepare for the worst, I'll just be stressed in anticipation. Much less gets done and with so much more anxiety. Am I rambling? I just need to calm my nerves.

My mother insisted on coming with me. I have to admit, her presence gave me strength. But you know what? It wasn't so bad. They attached several wires to Alex's chest with an adhesive. Not what you want to see, but Alex didn't seem uncomfortable. He watched a mobile for about two minutes and the test was over. The marvels of modern day magical medicine - that was all they needed. Results to come in a week.

By the way, Alex is still not sleeping through the night. We are getting up several times a night. I end up dealing with him but my husband still gets up every time the baby cries. The other kids- well they play musical beds throughout the night. They wake up and go into another bed or decide to sleep on the floor. I never know where I'll find someone in the morning. No one sleeps in our home.

Week Ten: Just Keep Living

The most important appointment this week is my phone call with Ethan's nutritionist. At the end of the call, I mentioned Alex's potential hearing loss and asked if there was anything nutrionally that could be beneficial.

It was a shot in the dark. I wasn't really expecting to get a positive response, but I did. Apparently, a few studies show that calcium and magnesium can help protect the ear from noise induced hearing loss. Since I was nursing, the nutritionist suggested I make sure that I at least have the recommended daily dose of calcium and magnesium. As it turns out, my prenatal vitamin did not have enough of either mineral. Since my diet was not heavy in calcium and my prenatal vitamin was deficient, it appeared that I did not have adequate calcium and magnesium.

She also suggested that I give Alex fish oil and that I should take fish oil supplements. Fish oil is shown to help with brain development. Babies are rapidly developing and her hope was that if a nutritional deficit caused the problem, proper nutrition could heal it. I was a little hesitant to give the oil directly to my little seven-week old baby, but after checking with my pediatrician, I decided to give him the daily drops.

You may be wondering why with all my positive experience with my nutritionist do I even bother to check anything with my pediatrician. That's a good question. In fact, my pediatrician has asked me the same question on several occasions. The conversation goes something like this:

With a sigh and a smile, "Haleh, does it matter what I tell you? You are going to do what you want anyway."

And I always respond. "Of course. You are a good person. You are good at what you do. I take what you say into consideration. I just might not always agree."

He shakes his head, smiles and answers whatever questions I have. Typically, the conversation ends with him handing me a script for a drug with the words, ". . . even though you are probably not going to use it. But I want to see you back in ten days." The truth is I respect him. He is knowledgeable in his chosen medical field. For me, he is my medical expert.

I have to give my mother credit. After I spoke with the nutritionist, I called my mom and gave her an update. The following is only a slight exaggeration: in the time it took me to hang up the phone, after my call with my mom, she had already gone shopping and was back ringing our doorbell. She had drops for Alex, vitamins for me, and a concoction of organic vegetables to make juices that would naturally provide the calcium and magnesium the nutritionist recommended. How'd she do that?

George arrived at two today. Who is George? Well, we need a dining room table. We have a large family and no place to seat guests. So, we have been on a quest. My husband happened to know a carpenter who offered to build us a table. Now the last thing I wanted to do was to talk to someone about decorating our home. We'd make do without having too many guests; with all that was going on, I thought a table could wait.

But my husband wanted to fix the situation. "It is what it is," he always says. "This is our life. We can't just stop living." So, I kept the appointment. George parked his pickup on our driveway and knocked on the door. He was a broad shouldered man, in jeans and working boots; he spoke in a deep voice. He stepped into our house carrying a stack of decorator's magazines. A little normalcy can go a long way in the middle of chaos. It was nice to think about something light for a change. But how I was to get to it was simply beyond me.

At six, I had an appointment for a new heater.

Wednesday is the day of Alex's MRI. My husband couldn't take off from work again, so my father insisted on coming with me. Though I resisted, I was later very glad that he came.

As with the sedated ABR, Alex again could not eat for several hours before the procedure. They needed to sedate him so that he would lie completely still during the test. I hoped that he would not need too much sedation. After the sedation for the ABR, his head just flopped around for a few hours before he had full control. Seeing that once was not the end of the world but I didn't want to see it again. It is such a milestone when babies hold up their heads that it felt like I was going backwards after one of these tests. I knew it was just a simple side effect that disappeared once the sedation fully wore off, but I didn't like it anyway.

As it turned out, he needed quite a bit of sedation to stop from fidgeting and crying. I had planned to sit in the room when they took the MRI. I stayed in there as they strapped Alex into the massive machine. I didn't think that my sedated baby looked peaceful. He looked defeated to me after fighting for so long not to fall asleep. Sedated, he couldn't even do the one thing babies do best- cry out.

Being in the room would be useless. I couldn't wear my glasses in the MRI room because of the metal in my frame- I just can't see without my glasses. To sit both literally and figuratively blind to all that was happening just made no sense. I needed a break. I stepped outside while they took their time magnetically looking into Alex's head for what felt like forever.

Outside, my dad tried to give me a pep talk. He hugged me and of course gave me some food to eat. Pep talks are only complete if accompanied by food. He said, "You know everything is fine. Don't worry. He will be okay. It's okay. He's okay. He'll be fine." He kept repeating. "He's okay. He's okay."

What I learned was that my dad was nervous. I was too drained to feel any anxiety myself. I tried to calm my dad down. I told him to please sit down and eat. There was nothing to worry about. But I did appreciate his hug. It's just that when I am concerned, worrying around me just makes things worse. On a deeper level, despite the difficulty, I think a part of me truly believed the mantra. I knew that God was with me and I was with God. I had the power and strength of God.

After the MRI, I picked up my floppy necked baby. When he was able to nurse, they released us. Boy was I glad my dad was with me. From here on, he took care of me. I didn't even remember where we parked the car. There was no way I could drive back home. I didn't have the strength. Besides, I needed to sit by Alex on the drive home and hold his head so that it would not excessively jostle around on the car ride back.

Thursday, the electrician came by. My in-laws had been over the weekend before and raised an issue that my husband and I had tried to ignore. The lights in our house did not always work. And they all seemed to burn out a little too quickly. And just recently, I discovered mouse dropping in the basement. Nowhere else, thankfully- but even that was pretty gross. In any event, the two were possibly linked. It was possible that mice were chewing on our wiring and we were just sitting on a fire hazard. I was no longer able to ignore the lighting issue.

I had an electrician over at the house. Guess what? No problem. Mice chewing wires applies to older homes which have cloth covered wiring. No fire hazard, but fixing our lighting problem could be costly, because it could be one of several different issues and take days to repair. Put the electrician on the back burner and continue poisoning the mice. (I hope I'm not offending any animal activists.)

Friday, one of my other sons complains of a stomachache after eating oats and chicken. Did I mention I had been to a pediatric gastroenterologist for him? He frequently complained of stomach pains; so, I have to keep track of what he eats and when. We'll see where this goes. It didn't seem like an emergency. By the way, I had another appointment for an estimate for the basement. Remember, my kids flooded it a few days before Alex was born. And so, life goes on. (Continued drinking the vegetable juice today)

Week Eleven: Drinking the Juice

Before I go into the particulars of this week, let me explain to you my food situation for the last few weeks. Remember the nutritional information I got and passed on to my mom? May God bless her, for I have no idea where she gets her energy. She spent the next three weeks at our home making sure that I drank several cups a day of various organic, raw vegetables all with the proper combination to ensure calcium and magnesium absorption into my body. After all, Alex would be getting my milk.

Her efforts were helping both Alex and me. My skin was simply amazing from this vegetable diet – it was glowing and youthful (if I do say so myself). In the midst of all of the chaos and difficulty at home, anyone who saw me out of the house would comment how wonderful I looked. Looks can be deceiving. My body was in great shape now and my eczema had completely disappeared. Of course, there was the side effect of a little nausea after each cup of juice. My body seemed to have trouble adjusting to this barrage of healthy food. And the stuff just tasted horrible. But I truly believed that Alex would be cured of his hearing loss. That is why I did it.

Monday morning at eight-thirty, right after the other kids were all set for school, Alex had to take a blood test. This is probably one of the hardest things for me to do with my babies. Who wants to see their little arms all wrapped in that stretchy rubber contraption with a needle going in to take their blood? I can't believe these little guys even have any to spare. But it is a necessity. So we took the blood test. He cried. I cried. By ten o'clock with a sleeping Alex, I was with my son's class volunteering to help in the library. Life moves on and everyone needs attention. Drink vegetable juice.

Tuesday, one of my sons goes to the doctor for his yearly checkup and the school needs a copy of his shots to make sure that he is up to date. They didn't have them yet and the nurse was giving me extra time to hand it in. Drinking the juice- doesn't my mom get tired of making it?

Wednesday, I had to go to the children's school at twelve-thirty to help out. Also, I had to call George for the table to let him know what I liked from the magazines he dropped off. I am still drinking several cups of green, bitter vegetable juice. Apparently, mixing any fruit into it is not good according to my mom. I mean it would taste great but if the stomach prefers not to mix fruits and vegetables together, who am I to argue? Besides, I think that Alex's hearing will be absolutely perfect when we retest in a month.

Hey, guess what? It's Thanksgiving Weekend. Usually we go to my husband's uncle's house for the holiday. This year, I am exhausted. There was no way I could make it; thankfully, my husband agreed. For the first time, we stayed home. Both my husband and I get some well-needed rest during the day. Still, no sleeping at night. Does anyone sleep at night?

Third Month: Can You Hear Me?

It's December now. Still drinking the vegetable juice. Starting to starve. Anyway, Alex is three months old. How does this happen? How can we do it? Wisdom comes with experience and age. I love children. Anyone whose life is touched by caring for others is forever changed. The lessons we learn leave us enriched. Okay, and sleep deprived.

Anytime someone asks me about having more kids my response is "go for it." Have another. Have two, have four. The more the merrier. But ultimately, we all get what we can handle. Not one too many and not one too few. Each person has a different path in life. What we choose to do with what we are given is what makes the difference.

Our hands are full with typical and not so typical issues facing our children. Money? Our need for it is limitless. Help? We can always use more. Values?

We're trying to teach them. Will actions alone transmit them? Love? I think it's here somewhere.

It is time for Alex's three-month ABR. I spend a couple of nights before the ABR throwing up. Oh, yes, it was back. After the birth of one of my children I started to have a problem. Periodically, I would spend the night in the bathroom throwing up. No apparent cause was ever found. Well, it was back again and this time with a vengeance. Normally, I would feel fine the next morning. Now it hung over me the next day. Masking my stress has a calming and positive affect on others, but it's not so good for me. These days, I could not exercise or take a moment for myself. I knew that it was all stress induced. But, since the nausea lasted longer, I felt compelled to make a round of appointments for myself just to make sure that all was well.

Alex couldn't eat for three hours prior to the sedated ABR. But by now, I was a pro at this. My husband and I sit patiently, as Alex falls asleep in the dark room and is once again hooked up with all the wires.

The audiologist starts the testing. The usual re-adjusting of wires and typing resumes. This time I am absolutely positive that the vegetable juices that I have been drinking, the daily calcium and magnesium and fish oil that I consumed and the fish oil that I give Alex, will show that his hearing is perfect. I was wrong.

He showed up with moderate to severe hearing loss in both ears. How could this be? There is no one in either of our families with a problem like this. It made absolutely no sense. HE CAN HEAR. I want to shout at the audiologists. Instead, I just asked questions. Why the change in three weeks? What is the reason? Why can't you explain it? Is it genetic? Can it be nutritional? What alternative remedies have you heard of? What *can* he hear? Can he hear a school fire alarm? Does he need hearing aids? Can he outgrow this? Will he speak normally? Will he hear like me with hearing aids? Where do I get them? Who can help?

I'll spare you the rest but I did not stop asking questions. I asked questions for the rest of the appointment. My husband didn't ask anything. There was nothing left to ask. A large part of my questioning was because I thought his hearing was fine. I had other children and was not exactly a novice. I knew he was actually hearing, and not following hand movements or simply responding to vibrations. But the audiologist patiently explained that I was just seeing what I wanted to see and that I was wrong because the test was right. She repeated empathetically that Alex needed hearing aids as soon as possible, before he was six months of age, if we wanted him to speak normally.

What if she was right? I needed to contact the early intervention program in my state for children with disabilities. I had to contact PHIR to enroll him and our family in a special program for the hearing impaired. I needed to get a social work appointment, a genetic testing appointment, and begin speech therapy. I had to contact hearing aid vendors. I had to call insurance to see what was covered. I had to contact organizations that provide services to parents with hearing impaired children.

I had to start watching videos and reading about how to teach our hearing impaired child to speak. I had to contact support groups. I had to seek out alternative remedies. I had to get a second opinion.

I walked out of there with the weight of the world on my shoulders. By the way, did you see how many times I use the word I? I I I I I I I I I I I. You see, it didn't matter that my husband was there with me. It didn't matter that my mother and father were helping me. It didn't matter that we have family and friends. This was primarily *my* burden and *my* responsibility. How could I possibly delegate the work required? Only I had been to *all* the doctor's appointments and knew what questions to ask and what needed to be done. And on top of everything with Alex, I still have the other children.

We came home. I spent the rest of the week on the phone. I couldn't care for my other children beyond the basic homework check. My mom cooked for us and took the kids to and from their different activities. In addition to making numerous appointments, I spoke to countless audiologists through an early intervention program as well as organizations aimed at helping the hearing impaired. I recounted Alex's test results and my experience with him and every single time the answers to my barrage of questions were the same. "PHIR is always right. The test results are accurate. There is nothing you can do. You are in denial. You will accept in time."

This mantra was very difficult to hear and hard to accept. Was it maternal instinct, was it the guiding hand from above, or was I just in denial? In any event, after every call, the wind was blown out of me. They forced me to face an inevitability of Alex's hearing loss. Though I knew logically that things could be worse, I only wanted Alex to hear the world like I did. Every night I was exhausted.

Christmas week was a blessing for me. It saved my life. Since most offices are closed and no one is around, I couldn't get anything done, what a blessing. Who says miracles don't happen anymore? This timing gave me a break that kept me from collapsing.

The nutritional route was not the only avenue we turned to for help. As soon as Alex was diagnosed with a hearing loss, my parents made sure his name was given to every religious institution in the area. People were praying for him everywhere. On New Year's Day, my parents took him to a very holy woman who prayed for Alex's health and hearing.

While we didn't have any doctor appointments this week, I didn't exactly take the week off. All week long the kids and I tested Alex's hearing non-stop. I could tell you what sounds he liked and disliked. I could tell you the distance from which he could hear sounds and at what volume. I could tell you that this child could hear. Why were my test results so different than the doctor's? Was I just hearing what I wanted to hear?

By the end of the month, Alex and I started speech therapy. You might be wondering, why does a baby who can't speak need speech therapy? Well, if a person has significant hearing loss, speech becomes very difficult to acquire. But speech is a fundamental communication tool for people. Even those who can barely hear what it is that everyone is talking about still need to express their ideas to others. I wanted my son to find a way to speak regardless of how much the doctors claimed he could hear.

Alex was part of this world. He needed to learn how to speak even if he could barely hear a thing. As a first lesson, babies need to learn that there is such a thing as "sound" that they need to focus on. Specialized speech therapists start by teaching babies to pay attention to the slightest sounds in their environment. The next steps involve teaching parents to speak with expression, in the direct vision of babies, and to speak with signs to help children make the connection between speech and the world around them. Most importantly, babies who are hard of hearing, in particular, need constant exposure to speech, since it requires more effort on their part to acquire it. The speech therapy was as much for Alex as it was for me to learn how to work with him.

But the most important thing that I learned during speech therapy was that maybe I wasn't imagining things. The speech therapist was the first person outside of our family who spent significant time with Alex. She was truly taking the time to get to know

Alex and address my concerns. Of course, I asked her all the questions that I'd asked everyone else. She answered everything she could and told me when a question was beyond her field of knowledge. She was objective and not driven by an emotional attachment to Alex. While it was not clear whether Alex responded to all sounds equally, it quickly became very clear that he was aware of various sounds at extremely low volumes, which he shouldn't be if he had moderate to severe hearing loss. The therapist, like me, was puzzled by Alex's diagnosis. Maybe I wasn't just hearing what I wanted to hear.

Keeping Track of it All

- Maintain a file with copies and results of all medical tests.
- Keep an accurate record of any alternative treatments and traditional methods of healing you are pursuing.
- Organize files by doctor or ailment as necessary (accordion file folders with multiple compartments can be helpful)
- Have with you contact information of all your doctors.
- Keep a list of all medications including alternative supplements that you use. (In an emergency, you may not be able to recall it all)
- Get out that old-fashioned paper monthly calendar that allows a single glance view of which days are already booked with appointments. This

way, if possible, you can try to create "breaks" in the hectic schedule.
- When dealing with children, teach them the names of medications and the frequency with which they need them. Although you may not yet be able to fully trust your child, this will begin the process of self-responsibility.
- If there is too much for you to organize, ask for help.

Fourth Month: It Takes Guts

His hearing aids arrived. We had a choice of several colors. We chose the flesh colored one; we thought it would be less obvious. As he got older, he could decide if he wanted another color. To everything new we must adjust. But what do you do when you have to adjust to something that just feels so wrong? I guess we do it because we have to. Medicines and their side effects can be difficult to manage – so can a little piece of equipment. Why do we accept it all? We believe in the science of medicine. We've been trained to believe that doctors know best.

Now, in my hand I held these hearing aids - tiny marvels of modern technology. And how fortunate that Alex could be diagnosed at such a young age and could then be taught to speak normally. But what if they were wrong? What if they were right? The problem was that I was unsure.

PHIR has a comprehensive program for children diagnosed with hearing problems. They recommend speech therapists, audiologists and counselors to help parents and patients adjust. My husband and I attended a counseling session together.

We walked into a cozy room with a large window. There were two overstuffed chairs for us to sit in. The room was small but we found a way to fit in Alex's stroller. The therapist had a warm smile and a welcoming manner. I got the distinct feeling from her that she truly cares and wants to help. We expressed our concerns and questioned the test results. The therapist's response?

"When faced with such a diagnosis, it is part of the normal grieving process for the loss of hearing to deny it and search for answers. But it is important that you provide your child with hearing aids so that he can hear," she explained calmly.

I responded, "Please, we have no issue with a hearing loss. Of course, we'd rather that he did not have one. But there are so many worse problems. The issue here is that we just don't think the diagnosis is correct. First, he appears to be hearing us and second, he had a sudden unexplained change in his hearing, as indicated by the ABR. Is this test accurate? Have you ever confronted this issue? Is there any way we can help him overcome this diagnosis, if correct?"

Again, with utmost patience, she continued, "I grew up with family members with hearing loss. I have been in this line of work for many, many years. What you are hoping for is not impossible but highly unlikely. Do what you have to become comfortable with this, but don't take too much time. You don't want to affect your child's ability to speak. Alex can only hear conversational level volume only within around four feet of himself and even that will not be clear for him. Here, let's listen to a tape of how Alex perceives the world at his level of hearing loss."

After listening to the tape, my heart sank. It was practically inaudible. Could this truly be all that Alex could hear? Yet, my husband and I knew after listening to that tape that Alex could hear better than what the tests showed. He was a highly interactive and aware baby, smiling and playing with anyone who showed him the slightest attention. We didn't understand how that would be possible if his hearing was so minimal. We expressed this to the counselor.

She repeated with understanding, "You have to do what you have to do to become comfortable with this diagnosis." We were not receiving any support from her for our doubts, but at least she was more polite than others had been. I had been hearing this same information in all my phone calls but said with much greater force and filled with explanations to allay my lack of ability to understand. "At least she was nice about it," I said to my husband, but he disagreed.

"She was condescending. She wasn't listening to a word we were saying. She had her own agenda and a prewritten script. She didn't seem to understand that there could be exceptions. She's just treating us like a statistic."

How would he have reacted if he had dealt with all the people I spoke to on a daily basis? Would he have been bullied into agreeing with them? Would he have given up? Would he have slammed down the phone and not bothered to follow up with anything? Would he have continued searching?

I tried to be a good parent and patient. I learned to clean the hearing aids. I could check the miniscule batteries and change them. I even learned to lean on the rest of the family. After all, we were all in it together. So we all learned to put the hearing aids back in his ears every time he took them out. We explained what was going on to the kids. We answered their questions. The older children were upset with the diagnosis. The younger kids didn't understand it. No one liked the hearing aids.

Every morning I put both hearing aids in his ears, and every day throughout the entire day, Alex just ripped them out. He winced when there was a loud noise but we were told Alex just was getting used to sounds that he could not hear before. It drove me crazy when he would take them out of his ears and start eating them. Hearing aids are small and they have small parts. I worried about him choking. But

I was told that his behavior would last only until he got used to them.

The stress of constantly putting the hearing aids in his ears was simply too much for me. I started to keep them in for only an hour a day when no one else was around so that I could keep my eyes focused on him. The home was pretty silent at that point. I am not sure what he got out of them but at least I could monitor that he would not eat them. Feeling badly that he wasn't wearing the hearing aids enough, I hired a babysitter to sit with him and watch him when the other kids were home. Alex cried and fussed the entire time. I stopped with the sitter.

I followed every direction: checking hearing aid batteries, cleaning the hearing aids, going back and forth to the audiologist to make sure that the ear molds fit properly. In little babies they need to be refitted sometimes every other week, because babies are constantly growing. I hated these hearing aids. They were so much work.

But I had to make peace with them. How could I not appreciate a piece of equipment that would help my son hear? Keeping these hearing aids in his ears was necessary in order for Alex to speak properly. But it just didn't feel right.

A friend suggested that we see a particular chiropractor that he knew. We did. Again, I drove out of town. This office was more like a spa than a medical office. Candles burned as soft music filled the space, the walls were painted honey colored brown and a few large plants flanked the corners of the spacious room.

This chiropractor wore a dress and had her long hair pulled back in a loose ponytail. I had the feeling that maybe I had traveled back to the sixties but without the tie-dye and with a modern sense of style. She gently adjusted Alex's spine to ensure that there would be proper energy flow in his body. I was told this would help him recover from the shock of birth and heal any problem he may have with his hearing. The first time she saw Alex she said, "You don't know me, but let me tell you, this baby is fine. There is nothing wrong with him." I liked her right away. We returned for several visits. I don't know what she was doing. I don't know if she helped him or gave me hope.

Another friend of ours has had hearing aids in both ears since he was three years old. He said: "If it was my kid, I wouldn't put on the hearing aids. You have to wait until he tells you what he can hear. When the audiologist tries to determine my hearing with only an ABR, and without actually asking me what I can hear, they are always wrong. They always put the hearing aids on louder than I need it. They don't know. Get a second opinion."

I protest, "But I am at PHIR - one of the best in the country."

"Get a second opinion," he says. Well, I thought I was getting second opinions all day long. After spending hours on the phone, I had consulted with numerous audiologists who all read his results in the same way. PHIR itself has several ENTs. But my questions had not been answered. No one had explained the change in test results from a child with hearing loss in one ear to a child with severe hearing loss in both ears or our observation that he seemed to be hearing fine. We decided to pursue yet another opinion.

In the meantime, life just marched on. Alex still had to be taken to have his eyes checked as part of the series of tests that was now required and he still had his normal monthly pediatric appointments. I was also going through a series of meetings with our State's early intervention program. The other kids had dentists, allergists and their normal checkup appointments. For a healthy family, the number of doctor's appointments boggled the mind. It is unimaginable to me what families go through who have even more serious conditions. The other kids still had school, after school activities and sleep-overs with their friends. For about two months my in-laws came down every other week to do our food shopping. I had absolutely no time to even go to the store.

Anyone who saw Alex wearing his hearing aids was very kind. I actually thought that people were nicer to him and played with him more. Not so bad for the youngest of a busy household.

It was a Friday morning. I dropped Ethan off at pre-school, and was once again going to the audiologist for *another* fitting of the ear molds. On my way there, Alex had of course taken out his hearing aids and begun chewing on them. Composed is not the way someone would describe my appearance or state. I was absolutely exhausted as the audiologist refitted Alex. I asked again if he really needed them. "Yes, he really needs them. You are doing great. You are a wonderful mom. You've done everything you can for him. This is not going to hurt him. It will only help him." It was nice to be told I was wonderful; but I felt defeated, being forced to accept something I felt was wrong.

After the appointment, I picked up Ethan from pre-school and went home. It so happened that my father walked in the door. He had the day off. He walked in and I walked out.

I had absolutely no idea what I was doing or where I was going. At some point, I decided to pull over and park. Being the rebel that I am, I was approximately half a mile away from home. But hey, just walking out was a big deal for me. It was pouring rain and I was crying nonstop. I cried from the pressure. I cried from the unfairness. I cried for being unthankful. I cried just to cry and then I fell asleep.

Here is how life imitates art. When I woke up, it had stopped raining. You know in the movies, the big symbolic turning point is always water or rain. It's so cliché but every movie has it. And now so did my life. Here's the next bit. I often listen to a radio show by Dennis Prager, to keep my mind active. Every Friday afternoon on his show, he has the "Happiness Hour". I am not sure if this particular happiness topic applied to me but tuning into the "Happiness Hour" after I had just been rained on felt like a message that all would be well. But I wasn't quite ready to go back home.

I am not sure if it is my personality or how everyone feels when their child has a health problem but Alex's hearing issue felt to me to be my burden more than anyone else's. At the end of the day, no matter how helpful everyone around me was, I was the one who took him to ninety-five percent of the doctor's appointments. I was the one who made the phone inquiries and, as a stay at home mom, I was the one who would have to adjust most to raising a hearing impaired child. He wasn't my only child. I had other children and Ethan's allergies still. I felt such a burden and such an inability to take care of myself, since everything else around me seemed so much more important.

I had a late lunch. I finally used a gift certificate that I had been carrying around for a local salon and got a massage and cut my long hair short. I went shopping and bought a new outfit. I "ran away" for about eight hours and then I went home.

My husband, parents, and brother were all waiting for me. The kids were asleep when I returned. I think I shocked my parents the most; they were extremely worried. My husband was happy that I took the break. My brother burst out laughing when he heard that I ran off. Thanks to him, they had been tracking me all around town through my credit card purchases.

I felt wonderful when I returned. I learned how important it is to take care of myself as a mother. I can be no good to anyone, if I burn out. With the help and understanding of my mother and husband, I returned to exercising once again.

Nurture Yourself: We Need Each Other

- Lean on friends, family and clergy for support.
- Take a break. Even something as short as a routine coffee break with a friend or walk around your neighborhood can help reenergize and focus.
- If possible, get away even if it's only for a weekend.
- Laugh often. Leave the tear-jerker movies for another time.
- Ask a friend or family member to come with you to an appointment, if you are anxious about possible test results.
- Contact support groups with others in your circumstance.

- Treat yourself to that extra haircut or little something. Those few dollars will go a long way.
- Get in the habit of hugging. Physical touch is therapeutic.
- Remember, better to take care of yourself now than to pay the far steeper cost in the future of your own ill health.
- Start your day recounting your blessings and being thankful.

Fifth Month: The Second Opinion

You have to wonder in life whether things happen by luck or if there is something larger at work. When I started to research where to go for a second opinion, a number of top institutions came up. Of course PHIR was one of them but there were several in New York and in other places around the country. Then someone gave my husband the name of an ENT in Boston. I researched the name. The doctor seemed promising and she was affiliated with one of the top institutions in the country. Her focus was on the hearing impaired and she was a researcher. After speaking to her assistant, I found that she was open to alternative remedies. Plus, she had an appointment available within two weeks.

Two weeks? Typically, you are lucky to get an appointment that is two months away. Now, Boston is considerably further from our home than New York

(Remember, New York, the center of the world?). This would require us to stay over night but she seemed okay and had an appointment right away. I was getting tired of researching everything to death, so we just went.

The appointment was on a Monday morning. We drove up Sunday night during the Super Bowl. The ride was easy. We found an excellent hotel right off the highway. It was beautiful. If you can believe, it was a little get-away in the middle of all the chaos. The next morning we found the doctor's office easily.

While we waited for the doctor we looked around the packed room at all the children. Many had hearing aids and some had cochlear implants. They were all normal kids who instead of glasses had something to help them hear. We sat for a long time. I kept checking my files making sure that I had copies of all of Alex's tests with me. The wait was worth it. I would wait for this doctor for hours if we had to.

The doctor actually listened. She listened patiently as we explained everything and then she asked questions as she read through Alex's file with us. She spent an hour with us. She acknowledged that the test results were odd and actually believed me when I told her that Alex could hear. Unlike the many doctors who I spoke to in person and over the phone, she did not treat me as if I was in denial over a foregone conclusion. She respected that I continued to question the unusual test results. She praised the "alternative" approach of giving him fish oil. Apparently, this was on the forefront of cutting edge research, in which she was involved. Fish oil helps with brain development and could help with certain hearing issues- especially the diagnoses she suspected- auditory neuropathy.

Essentially, she said that Alex's ear functioned normally but the nerves, which send auditory messages to the brain, were not fully developed. This is sometimes seen in pre-mature babies, which Alex was not. Parents of children with this diagnosis may report that their children appear to hear normally.

Auditory neuropathy is a spectrum disorder. On one end of the spectrum, children require surgery and cochlear implants in order to have any hearing.

On the other end of the spectrum, children hear normally. And in between lies everything from difficulty in hearing with background noise, to hearing sounds jumbled together, to many other various forms of interference in perceiving sound. We did not know where Alex lay in the spectrum.

Since Alex's extensive medical testing showed that he did not have any other issues, Alex was in the group of babies who could outgrow this by the time he reached one and half. With this diagnosis, rather than helping Alex, the hearing aids would permanently harm his hearing. The amplified volume of the hearing aids would actually cause loss of normal hearing function, and result in needing hearing aids. The PHIR doctors immediately agreed with this diagnosis.

I was surprised by the reaction I received from the PHIR doctors. My expectation was that they would apologize and acknowledge the mistake they made. Instead they simply agreed with the new diagnosis as if they knew it all along. As an attorney, I reasoned that perhaps they were afraid of a lawsuit;

though there was no actionable cause of action. In the end, Alex was never harmed by their misdiagnosis. We stopped using the hearing aids before he lost any hearing due to the constant unnecessary loudness. As a parent, I was upset.

When I pointed out that they made a mistake, they simply said, "You know Alex is an exception, this is not how it normally goes."

I pressed and suggested that perhaps this information should be shared maybe he is not such an exception. They said, "We don't want to raise anyone's hopes unnecessarily. Most cases don't turnout this way. We don't want parents not to use hearing aids when it is necessary."

This time I protested, as I spoke to the audiologist, "The problem is that you never even listened to me or evaluated the unusual change in test results he had."

The response blew me away. "I've never seen a doctor write so much in the file about a case. Clearly he thought about this case. I even brought up Alex at a conference I recently attended. I never saw a case like this."

At this point I just dropped it. PHIR was also perplexed by Alex. But why did it appear that they never listened or even acknowledged that I had a point when I questioned the test results? Why did they seem to mock any attempt at seeking other possible treatments? Doctors are trained in medicine not communication.

Over the next couple of years, I continued with speech therapy for Alex. He was always within normal range of speech development but because of his diagnosis, it was necessary to keep him under watch to see what, if any, auditory processing problems he had.

During this time, my mom happened to be reading several books on the importance of proper nutritional and hormonal balance, which included information about the effect of fish oil on brain development. My mom contacted the scientist who wrote the books to inquire about how this could help Alex. As a result, I changed the type and increased the dosage of fish oil Alex had. And within one week, he showed significant and dramatic improvements in speech, surpassing speech development standards for his age.

Today, Alex is bilingual and has normal expressive language development and normal hearing tests in the sound booth. Was it due to the chiropractor? Was it due to the additional nutritional support of the fish oil? Was it due to the calcium and magnesium supplements or vegetable juices that I had? Was it the prayers? Would he simply have outgrown it? All of the above?

Conclusion

I shared the hecticness and pain of our lives with you for a reason. We are all the same. We are all busy. We all face adversity. And while we want most to trust the opinions of professionals, we need to stay sharp.

I am thankful that I did not stop looking for treatments and answers. It is draining to continue questioning doctors whose expertise, knowledge and training lead many of them to believe that their approach and understanding is complete. It is exhausting to pursue different remedies. It is unsettling to always be in a state of doubt.

Being open to all possibilities, constantly questioning and continually hoping lead to positive results. To the extent that we are successful in creating partnerships with our medical doctors, it can only be more helpful. Ethan could've been a child living off formula with numerous developmental and emotional issues. Instead, he is healthy and thriving. Alex could've been a child with severe hearing loss who wears hearing aids or has a cochlear implant and requires significant therapy to facilitate speech development. Instead, he is developing normally.

We never know what is in store for us. It is the approach we take in life and what we demand from life that alters how we travel and what path we take. It is true that our ultimate fate is not in our hands but it is incumbent upon us to strive for a life that we can live to its fullest. May you be blessed with the wisdom and strength to unleash your fullest potential for a healthy and rich life.

P.S. At the time of this writing, we still don't have a dining room table. I am hopeful that in time, this too will remedy itself. But we have succeeded in evicting the mice from our basement. We are now a mice free home.

Discussion / Reading Group Questions

1. Could you relate to the mother? Did you feel that you could connect to the characters?
2. When Alex was ten days old, the parents went to PHIR concerned about his circumcision, which turned out to be fine. The author writes, "Little did I know, he was going to repeat this pattern." Do you believe that in life, there are patterns into which we fall?
3. Do you think that the mother came to help her children because she was in denial or do you think that she was able to help them because she refused to accept the situations?
4. Recalling the incident of the child with a peanut allergy who came to this mother's home, would you feel comfortable sending your child with allergies to her home?

5. Have you ever disagreed with your doctor's diagnosis? What did you do about it?
6. What do you think about "testing" alternative methods on yourself or your child, which have not been scientifically proven in the United States?
7. What are techniques that you have used to help a child deal with illness?
8. To what extend do you think frame of mind affects the healing process?
9. Do you think that there is a communication gap between patients and doctors? If you do, what do you think is the cause?
10. Are there times when you think questioning doctors and searching for alternative solutions could actually be harmful?

PLEASE SHARE YOUR STORY WITH ME

Go to: www.littlepatientbigdoctor.com

Some Books I've Read

The Anti-Aging Zone, Barry Sears, Ph.D.

Beginner's Guide to Reiki, David F. Vennells

The Cure Within: A History of Mind-Body Medicine, Anne Harrington

The Dynamic Laws of Prosperity, Catherine Ponder

Enzymes for Autism and other Neurological Conditions, Karen DeFelice

How Doctors Think, Jerome Groopman, M.D.

How To Talk So Kids Will Listen & Listen So Kids Will Talk, Adele Faber and Elaine Mazlish

If You Were God, Aryeh Kaplan

Natural Relief for Your Child's Asthma, Steven J. Bock, M.D., Kenneth Bock, M.C. and Nancy P. Bruning

Siblings Without Rivalry, Adele Faber & Elaine Mazlish

Made in the USA
Lexington, KY
30 December 2010